LEARNING
ABOUT EPILEPSY

The author's work on this book was made possible through a grant entitled "Improved Care of the Institutionalized Epileptic Person," funded by the Department of Health, Education, and Welfare, Region III, 1974–1976.

LEARNING ABOUT EPILEPSY

William B. Svoboda, M.D.
Associate Professor of Pediatrics and Neurology
West Virginia University Medical Center
Morgantown, West Virginia

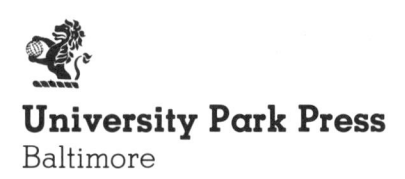

University Park Press
Baltimore

UNIVERSITY PARK PRESS
International Publishers in Science, Medicine, and Education
233 East Redwood Street
Baltimore, Maryland 21202

Copyright © 1979 by University Park Press

Composed by University Park Press, Typesetting Division.
Manufactured in the United States of America by
The Maple Press Company

All rights, including that of translation into other languages, reserved. Photomechanical reproduction (photocopy, microcopy) of this book or parts thereof without special permission of the publisher is prohibited.

Library of Congress Cataloging in Publication Data

Svoboda, William B.
Learning about epilepsy.

Includes index.
1. Epilepsy. 2. Epilepsy in children. I. Title.
RC372.S94   616.8'53   79-14639
ISBN 0-8391-1380-3

Contents

Preface and Acknowledgments ix

1 PREVIEW 1
The Frustration and the Response 1
The Overall Problems of Epilepsy 2
The Challenge 6

2 DEFINITION 9
Definition of a Seizure 9
Stages of a Seizure 9
What's Happening in the Brain During the Seizure 13

3 TYPES OF SEIZURES 17
Classification 17
Focal Seizure Disorders 18
Generalized Seizure Disorders 25
Unilateral Seizure Disorder 29
Multifocal — Mixed — Seizure Disorders 30
Neonatal (Newborn) Seizures 30
Unclassified Seizure Disorders 31
Applied Classification 31

4 CAUSES OF SEIZURES 35
Inherited Seizure Problems 35
Mixed Seizure Causes 36
Idiopathic and Acquired Seizure Disorders 36
The Types of Seizures 37
Timing and Circumstances of the Seizure Problem 38
Age of Onset of the Seizure Problem 40
The Course of the Seizure Disorder 41

5 EXAMINING THE PATIENT 45
History 45
The Examination 47

6 MIMICS OF SEIZURE DISORDERS 57
Peculiar Behaviors, Disturbed Emotions, or
    Strange Thoughts 58
Sensory Symptoms, Sometimes with Headaches 60
Staring Episodes 61
Loss of Consciousness 62
Abnormal Movements: Jerks, Stiffening, or Falling 62

vi   Contents

7 LABORATORY DIAGNOSIS 67
Hospitalization 67
Levels of Diagnostic Studies 68
Basic Studies... 69
Follow-Up Studies 79
Further Studies That May Be Risky 81
Supplemental Studies 83

8 ACUTE SEIZURE MANAGEMENT 93
Types of Acute Seizure Attacks 93
Dangers of Long or Frequently Recurring Seizures 94
Management of Acute Seizures 95
Why Did the Seizure Occur? 101

9 ONGOING ANTICONVULSANT MANAGEMENT 103
Beginning Therapy 103
Adjusting the Medicine 109
Special Situations.. 111
Addition of a Second or Even a Third and Fourth Drug 113
Substitution of One Drug for Another 116
Withdrawal: Gradually Discontinuing a Drug..................... 116

10 ANTICONVULSANT SIDE EFFECTS 121
Intoxication 121
Allergies 125
Idiosyncratic Reactions 129
Risks with Pregnancy 131

11 OTHER APPROACHES TO SEIZURE MANAGEMENT 135
Managing Common Stresses of Life 135
Behavioral Approaches 143
Surgical Approaches 150
Other Approaches 152

12 EMOTIONAL AND BEHAVIORAL CONSEQUENCES OF EPILEPSY .. 157
Types of Problems... 157
Behavior Problems 158
Reactions... 159
Behavioral Responses 160
Dependence Versus Independence 163
General Management 163
Seizures and Psychiatric Disturbances........................... 164
Treatment of Emotional Disturbances 170
The Home 172
Institutionalization 177
Environment 178

13 EPILEPSY AND LEARNING PROBLEMS ... 185

Behavioral Interferences with Learning ... 186
Unrecognized Seizures ... 187
Speech Problems and Seizures ... 188
Specific Learning Disabilities ... 189
Depressed and Deteriorating Intelligence ... 194
Placement ... 195

14 RESTRICTIONS AND RESOURCES ... 201

Sports Activities ... 201
Other Activities ... 202
Driving Restrictions ... 203
Insurance ... 204
Dating, Marriage, and Family ... 204
Problems of Employment ... 204
Social Security Benefits ... 212
Resources for Help ... 214
Advocacy and the Law ... 219

15 THE FUTURE ... 223

Diagnosis ... 223
Response to Medications ... 223
Overall Outlook ... 225

APPENDIX: RESOURCES FOR FURTHER INFORMATION AND HELP ... 227

Index ... 233

Preface and Acknowledgments

The goal of this book is to present in simple terms a review of all that is needed in good management for any person with epilepsy. The patient and the family need to know all that can and should be done in good care so that they may seek it. The provider, whether a physician, a nurse, a teacher, a counselor, or some other professional, also needs to know so that he or she may, working together with others, provide the needed help. Everyone must keep in mind that there is no single, perfect method of management. Instead, I have tried to indicate at least one common method for each type of problem.

This text is largely built upon the questions, comments, problems, and needs of my patients, their families, students, nurses, teachers, counselors, other professionals, and the general public as I have worked with them and spoken with them. The effort began through the help of Mrs. Elizabeth Schoenfeld of HEW Region III, and was proposed under the encouragement of Mrs. Evelyn Bombay and the other capable members of the nursing staff of Colin Anderson Center for the Mentally Retarded. The sections on behavior and on learning mirror the help of two exceptional educational psychologists skilled in working with children who have epilepsy, Mrs. Diane Wangelin and Mrs. Marilyn Thatcher. Mrs. Barbi Slevin stimulated much of the section on vocational rehabilitation through her expertise as a counselor.

The book emerged under the simplifying and correcting eye of my wife Lois and my daughters Karen and Heather. It took final shape through the hard work of a series of dedicated secretaries, Barbie Slevin, Lois Cashdollar, Jane Nease, Susan Richards, Phyllis Haislip, Judy Pauley, and Kathy Keefover, all of whom not only typed, but also corrected, commented, and produced further questions to answer.

It is quite apparent that this book is a team effort, just as the care of the problems of epilepsy should be. This book is written for those who need to know and for those who want to know: our efforts are rewarded if the reader is able to develop better approaches as a result of the contribution of this team.

LEARNING
ABOUT EPILEPSY

1
PREVIEW

Since ancient times epilepsy has been a mysterious, misunderstood, and dreaded problem. For many centuries seizures were associated with demonic possession, religious ecstasies, and impure living. People looked to magic or to religion for cures (O'Leary and Goldring, 1976). Even today, mysticism, myth, and misunderstanding dominate attitudes toward epilepsy. The primary attitude seems to be "Ignore it; perhaps it will go away." Yet those suffering with, living with, and working with epilepsy realize the need for a positive approach, a "What can be done to help?" attitude, if anything is to be accomplished. This concern is the first step toward conquering the problems of epilepsy.

THE FRUSTRATION AND THE RESPONSE

By the early 1970s, the frustrations of the patients, their families, and dedicated workers in the field had begun to unite in a cry for help. The federal government responded with the creation of the Commission for Control of Epilepsy and Its Consequences, which was mandated to spend nearly two years in an exhaustive, detailed study of the medical and social implications of epilepsy in the United States. Practically no stone was left unturned. The core of specialists drawn from differing fields was directed not just to conduct a fact-finding session; it was to identify both needs and current approaches being practiced; it was to develop specific recommendations as well as a national plan for the management of epilepsy and its consequences. This plan was to be based on and documented by a thorough study, including the gathering and interpretation of all available facts and figures. To broaden the approach, the commission itself called upon experts from a wide range of specialities and disciplines; it called for the active input of both complaints and ideas from the people closest to epilepsy...the patients and their families; it visited far and wide many different programs working with epilepsy. The picture that began to emerge was both shocking and disturbing, although not totally surprising to those already actively involved in the field of epilepsy. The final report discussed the problems identified below.

THE OVERALL PROBLEMS OF EPILEPSY

Epilepsy today is still a vague and misunderstood disorder. Voltaire advised, "If you wish to converse with me, define your terms." Science has not yet even reached this step in the understanding of epilepsy. Yet, if a problem is not defined clearly, if it is not understood, how can it be handled effectively? For centuries people have been satisfied by the mere diagnosis "epilepsy." Only recently has there been some attempt to classify epilepsy more specifically by using terms such as grand mal, petit mal, psychomotor, akinetic, myoclonic, and minor seizures. However, these terms often have been applied inconsistently, erratically, and with little agreement or documentation.

Epilepsy is not a single, simple syndrome of similar symptoms; it is a convenient collection of many very different types of seizures that vary widely in severity, appearance, cause, consequence, and management. A clear, common, and consistent classification has not been used uniformly, although one is now available (Gastaut, 1970).

In recent decades there has been an explosion of new treatment methods, of more effective management, and of improved diagnostic tools, both medically and in non-medical fields. Yet attempts to apply specific approaches to specific aspects of epilepsy have only revealed the flimsiness of the facts and figures on which we have been depending. It seems that the assumptions are based more on myths and magic than on scientific correlations and proofs. Currently accepted management methods at times seem more related to hopes, testimonials, and expert opinions than to tested, unbiased trials.

The educated public now wants statistics regarding the risks and probabilities of the appearance of certain problems as well as the chances of various outcomes. The specialist turns to his references, only to find that the specific facts are either vague or are not available. Statistics vary widely, depending on the source. Useful information is lost amid the confusion of conflicting facts and opinions. Often the consultant is too proud to say "We don't have the answer," and retreats to a reply consistent with his personal view, which tends to be a vague estimate and is as likely to perpetuate myths as it is to clarify the issue. When the experts cannot agree, the listener has real difficulties in understanding what they are talking about.

The commission experienced this problem again and again. Consequently, rather than exact facts and figures in documentation of their findings, they could only give good estimates obtained by comparing many sets of opinions and counter-opinions. They also were able to point out real needs for good definitions and exact classifications as a basis for exact scientific documentation of the values of various management approaches. They were able to indicate major problems that all specialists agreed upon, the needs that are indicated in this chapter (Commission for Control of Epilepsy, 1977).

Epilepsy Is a Social Stigma!

The word "epilepsy" comes from a Greek word meaning "to come upon, to be grabbed hold of or thrown down, to attack, to seize hold of." The term indicates truthfully that something overcomes the patient against his will; it does not describe what the attack looks like, its severity, its cause, or its associated problems. It is a label that, unfortunately, through the many centuries of being linked to demons, retardation, and strange behavior, has become socially unacceptable. The Biblical attitudes spill over into our modern life; we still feel that "epilepsy and leprosy are two disorders thou shalt not have." Society tends to exclude both disorders as being "unclean." Yet no more compassionate handling of the epileptic can be seen than that displayed by Jesus (see Mark 9:16-29, Luke 9:37-42). The label "epileptic" often proves to be more handicapping than the seizure itself.

It is probably wise in general not to talk about the disorder or to use the unacceptable word "epilepsy" unless necessary, especially when referring to a specific person. An alternative and indeed a more desirable approach is to use a more specific term if a label is needed. Yet this total avoidance of the term "epilepsy," as practiced by society in general and by specialists in particular, is nothing more than a throwback to the attitude of "Ignore it and it may go away" — it is to run away from the non-acceptance issue rather than to face it. If and whenever the word "epilepsy" can be used to bring people together, to stimulate movements on behalf of the epileptic, to develop hope rather than helplessness, to stimulate services and programs, to create positive awareness, or to generate financial support for movements, the label becomes a blessing rather than a curse.

Epilepsy Is a More Common Problem Than Is Thought

In a federal review in the year 1973, the estimated number of epileptic patients in the United States was greater than the combined sum of all of the cancer patients, all of the Parkinsonism patients, all of the cases of cerebral palsy, all of the multiple sclerosis (and related disorders) patients, all of the cases of the muscular dystrophies, all of the tuberculosis (and related lung disease) patients, all of the Huntington's chorea patients, and all of the myasthenia gravis patients. Yet it is these other diseases, much more than epilepsy, that attract national movements, major funding drives, and medical school emphasis (see "Neurological and Sensory Disabilities" in References).

By present estimates, about 1 of every 100 people in the United States has active epilepsy. This probably is an underestimate. There are a significant number of people that are unwilling to admit to their epilepsy because it may cause them to lose their jobs and friends. There are a significant number of undiagnosed epileptics. It is estimated that as many as 1 of every 4 epileptic patients are neither under medical care nor receiving the help of any social service agencies. In some rural areas, as many as 1 of every 5 cases of epilepsy has not been diagnosed.

In residential institutions, for example, the incidence of epilepsy has been grossly underestimated. In a study by the author and others involving one institution for the mentally retarded, the original estimate of the frequency of epilepsy was only around 12%. After a thoughtful reconsideration by the nursing staff in review of the charts and patients individually, the estimate was revised to around 33%. Then, after evaluation and a period of observation of suspected cases, the true incidence of epilepsy among this retarded population was determined to be at least 40%, with additional patients suspected (see "Approaches to Improved Care" in References).

The true incidence of epilepsy may be changing. Modern medical methods may be preventing the development of some cases of epilepsy. Yet similar techniques, such as those that are now utilized with improved obstetrical care, with the high-risk newborn programs, with intensified care for critical illnesses, and with modern trauma units, may be saving the lives of individuals who have suffered a sufficient degree of brain insult to place them at risk for later seizures. Head trauma from accidents adds thousands to the roster of epileptics yearly. Improved public understanding and acceptance, the removal of restricting laws against epileptics, and new hopes in more effective methods of treatment have persuaded many people to admit to their seizure problem.

Epilepsy Is Expensive

In the United States the annual cost of epilepsy is at least three billion dollars. Treatment costs are estimated at about one-third of a billion dollars or more per year. The average yearly cost of the medications alone for one person is more than $200. When one also considers the major expenses for the support of special education and rehabilitative services, for unemployment compensation, for hospitalization and institutional care, as well as the relatively small amount now spent for research for the epileptic, the costs mount up.

Epilepsy Is Not Only a Handicap, It Is Handicapping

Seizures are often not as handicapping as their associated problems. Roughly, 3 of every 4 epileptic individuals have multiple problems. Nearly half of the patients experience significant problems in learning. This is especially true with children. More than half of the patients have major emotional and behavioral difficulties. About 1 of every 10 epileptic people has some other significant neurologic problem, such as cerebral palsy. The patients and parents feel that the problems of education and employment, of emotional disturbances and behavior problems, and of social acceptance are far greater concerns than the seizures themselves. Travel and transportation, insurance, and the high costs of care and medication are additional considerations. A significant irritant to the patient and the family is the lack of concern, explanation, availability, and overall help from the experts.

Epilepsy is a negative influence on school performance: It may relate to problems in learning and behavior and to adjustment difficulties. These problems carry over into employment; here they are magnified by concerns over injury risks, productivity, and transportation to and from the job. Consequently the adult epileptic patient tends to be underemployed, unemployed, or, in some cases, unemployable.

As may be expected in light of the frequency of the frustrations and rejections the patient faces, a significantly high number of epileptic patients are emotionally disturbed. What is surprising is that a majority of the epileptic population has been able to live a relatively normal life.

Epilepsy Can Be a Threat to Life and Function

There is a tendency toward deterioration of mental, emotional, and behavioral function in the epileptic patient. Even more startling, though, is the estimate that nearly half of the epileptic population will die of conditions directly or indirectly related to their seizures. This figure includes deaths not only from the seizures themselves, and from seizure-related accidents and drownings, but also from suicides. The life expectancy of the epileptic may be reduced by as much as 10 years.

Epilepsy Is More Than an Individual Problem, It Is a Family Problem

At least half of the cases of epilepsy begin before adolescence; at least 75% of epilepsies appear before adulthood. The worries, frustrations, and problems experienced by the family of the epileptic patient are not fully appreciated. Their entire lifestyle may be altered radically. Interactions between family members often change drastically. The developing child and his siblings fall under the influence of this change.

Epilepsy Is a Problem of Many Kinds of Unmet Needs

The organization, interaction, coordination, and cooperation of real and potential services serving the epileptic patient at local, regional, state, and national levels are in a state of dispute and disarray. In the few situations where adequate information is available, those in need often do not know of it or are hesitant to seek it. The practicing physician is often not aware of modern medical breakthroughs in diagnosis and management methods; if he knows of them, he may not use them because of lack of time or training or disagreement with the recommendations. The frequent complications of learning disorders, emotional disturbances, behavioral difficulties, and social disturbances are usually not recognized or adequately managed when they are stumbled upon. Needed services are often not available; when they are available they tend to be unpublicized and thus under-utilized. Often a sea of red tape stands between the patient in need and the service. Specialists may consider referral to the service unnecessary, since they feel that as experts they can do better than others; more often, they are not aware of the service.

Little active research is being done about the means of delivering effective services. The few cases of such research projects, such as the project toward improving the care of the institutionalized epileptic patients, showed that markedly improved care can be developed, leading to improved control and functioning in the epileptic population.

Many of the problems clearly identified by the commission are common to other neurological disabilities and probably to many other medical disabilities in general. The efforts of the commission may lead to the development of more efficient and more effective care provisions in many areas in addition to that of epilepsy.

THE CHALLENGE

In August 1977 the Commission submitted its final report, a fact-packed, four-volume "Plan for Nationwide Action on Epilepsy." This alone is a major breakthrough. The observations quoted above show the increased awareness that this study has developed. If this vast collection of facts, figures, questions, and identified needs were all that had been produced, it still would be a major contribution as *the* reference on epilepsy. However, the commission went further: it identified successful programs dealing with the unmet needs, it suggested possible approaches toward better services and toward solving the problems identified in the study, it presented a picture of, and thus new standards for, what good care can and should be. The commission's efforts represent not only a major advance, but also a tool for change and improvement. The question no longer is "What is needed?" but rather "Why aren't we doing it?" The questioners are no longer the service-minded specialists, they are now the consumers, impatient for action and answers. Finally, the commission tried to suggest remedies to these well-documented needs by including 400 specific recommendations, including implementation strategies, cost estimates, and responsibilities, all aimed toward improving the management of epilepsy and its consequences.

Those experiencing epilepsy and those working with epileptic individuals now have a well-documented reference guide and a map to chart future possibilities. The report states what is and what is not known about epilepsy, what is available and what is needed, what has and what hasn't worked, what is being done, what can be done, and what should be done. It suggests what good care is, and how ideal care may be developed. The responsibility for pushing these recommendations to the stage of active application rests on the shoulders of each person experiencing or working with epilepsy.

To be successful and effective, those working with the epileptic individual must be aware of and be able to provide services within their areas of expertise. They must be aware of the potential contributions and services of other experts, and they must be able to talk with, work with, and refer to these other disciplines. They must be aware of what is being done, what can be done, and what should be done (and must be done) to help the epileptic patient. They must be willing to pursue these services whenever possible, so that the patient may benefit. In general, they must be able, alert, and active in 1) the early recognition of all the needs of the epileptic and his family, 2) the full remediation and rehabilitation of all problems they can manage, and 3) the appropriate referral for help for all needs beyond their particular skills.

To help launch the reader toward these goals, the succeeding chapters serve as a stepwise introduction to the basic aspects of epilepsy. Each chapter is followed by documenting references and further reading, appropriately identified, for more intensified study in specific areas. In the proper approach for medical personnel working with the epileptic patient, if there be any set rules, they would consist of four basic commandments:

I. You shall treat the whole patient, not just the seizure!
II. You shall treat the patient's needs, not just your own particular interests.
III. You shall treat as a team member, because no individual is able to know all or do all that is needed by the epileptic individual.
IV. You shall help others to treat the epileptic patient appropriately.

REFERENCES AND SUGGESTED READING

Approaches to Improved Care of Institutionalized Epileptic Persons: A collaborative project involving Region HEW III, performed under the direction of the Pediatric Seizure Clinic, John F. Kennedy University Affiliated Center, Johns Hopkins Hospital, Baltimore, Maryland, John M. Freeman, Director. Copies of this report may be obtained by contacting the Developmental Disabilities Training and Technical Assistance Center, c/o Ms. Muriel Rose, School of Social Work and County Plans, University of Maryland, 525 West Redwood Street, Baltimore, Maryland 21201. *(This report can serve as an excellent beginning guideline for those working with institutionalized epileptic persons. It is an outgrowth of a study on various approaches in management of such patients.)*

(The) Commission for Control of Epilepsy and Its Consequences. 1977. Plan for Nationwide Action on Epilepsy, 4 Volumes, Office of Scientific and Health Reports. National Institute of Neurological and Communicative Disorders and Stroke, Bldg. 31, Room 8A406, Bethesda, Md. 248 pp. (Vol. I.)

Gastaut, H. 1970. Clinical and electroencephalographical classification of epileptic seizures. Epilepsia 11:102-113. *(This is the recommended classification and the one that will be used throughout this text.)*

Neurological and Sensory Disabilities: Estimated Numbers and Costs. Report prepared by the Information Office, National Institute of Neurological Diseases and Stroke, National Institutes of Health, Bethesda, Md. Revised in 1973.

O'Leary, J. W., and S. Goldring. 1976. Science and Epilepsy. Raven Press, New York.

2
DEFINITION

DEFINITION OF A SEIZURE

Any brief, unusual action or behavior, such as the loss of consciousness, a stare, a short period of confusion, a recurring thought, a peculiar feeling, an emotional outburst, a strange sensation, an odd posturing, or uncontrolled movements, may be a seizure symptom.

STAGES OF A SEIZURE

Like any event, a seizure has a beginning, interval activities, and an ending. People usually see only a portion of the obvious attack, but they think that they have seen the entire seizure. Often they have not. Obvious symptoms, such as stiffening, jerking, or falling, are easily noted. Early symptoms, such as peculiar emotions or sensations, may be overlooked. The patient experiences these symptoms, but they are not obvious to the observer, who remains unaware of their existence.

The Build-up (or Prodrome)

Occasionally a patient may experience a gradual change in alertness, personality, emotions, or behavior for a period of hours to days before the main seizure occurs. The patient's family looks forward to the big seizure as the release valve, because when it finally occurs the patient reverts back to his usual self.

The Warning (or Aura)

The seizure may begin as a peculiar sensation, thought, fear, emotion, discomfort, or vague feeling. The symptom may be located in some specific part of the body or it may be diffuse and vague, as if it were felt all over the body. This warning-aura is the beginning of the attack. Sometimes the attack goes no further than these early symptoms. More often the attack continues to a more recognizable symptom, such as a jerk, a stiffening, a fall, or a loss of consciousness.

Noting the warning-aura symptoms is most important. The type of aura suggests where in the brain the seizure might be originating. The aura suggests that the seizure probably is a focal attack and not a generalized seizure problem.

To pinpoint the affected focal area, the neurologist keeps in mind a map of the brain and its different areas (see Figure 2.1). He considers the main functions of each area of the brain and compares them to the type of functional disturbances of the seizure onset.

As is shown in Figure 2.1, the brain is divided into five parts, or *lobes.* The front half of the brain (the *frontal lobe*) is large. Its lower under-surface seems to be related to the temporal lobe. The back part of the frontal lobe relates to movements of the opposite side of the body. In the very back part of the brain is the *occipital lobe,* which relates to visual functions. Between the frontal lobe and the occipital lobe, on the back half of the brain, is the *parietal lobe,* which handles various body sensations. On the lower sides of the brain, roughly in the brain area beneath the ear, is the *temporal lobe.* This complex area relates to memories, emotions, fears, and mistaken sensations. At the junction between the parietal and temporal lobe on the left brain half is located the area for understanding speech and reading. The upper part of the temporal lobe relates to hearing. The temporal lobe and the underneath portion of the frontal lobe seem to be related, handling thoughts, emotions, and fears. Between the lower part of the back portion of the frontal lobe and the upper part of the temporal lobe is a portion of the brain, the insula, which relates to movements and sensations of the mouth and abdomen. There are also portions of the brain on the medial surfaces between the two brain halves, and a part called the limbic system, which relates to tastes, smells, automatic acts, and autonomic nervous system reactions.

The warning-aura may involve the autonomic nervous system and its controls over the internal organs of the body. The patient might note spasms of the throat or mouth. He might complain of abdominal bloating, belching, strange rising sensations, butterflies in the stomach, thirst, vomiting, diarrhea feelings, or a vague abdominal discomfort. He may note discomfort in his chest, a feeling of a lack of air, or he may begin with irregular breathing. His heart rate may be fast, pounding, or irregular. He may appear pale or he may blush. He may complain of peculiar feelings or abnormal functions of the urinary or genital parts of the body. Such symptoms make the neurologist suspect that the attack may come from the medial portion of the temporal lobe, or occasionally from the deep nerve cells around the third ventricle, which is a natural cavity deep in the brain.

Other warnings may include burning, tingling, numbness, hot flashes, sensations of cold, shivering, heaviness, or the sense of movement in some area of the body. The location may be vague or quite specific. Sometimes

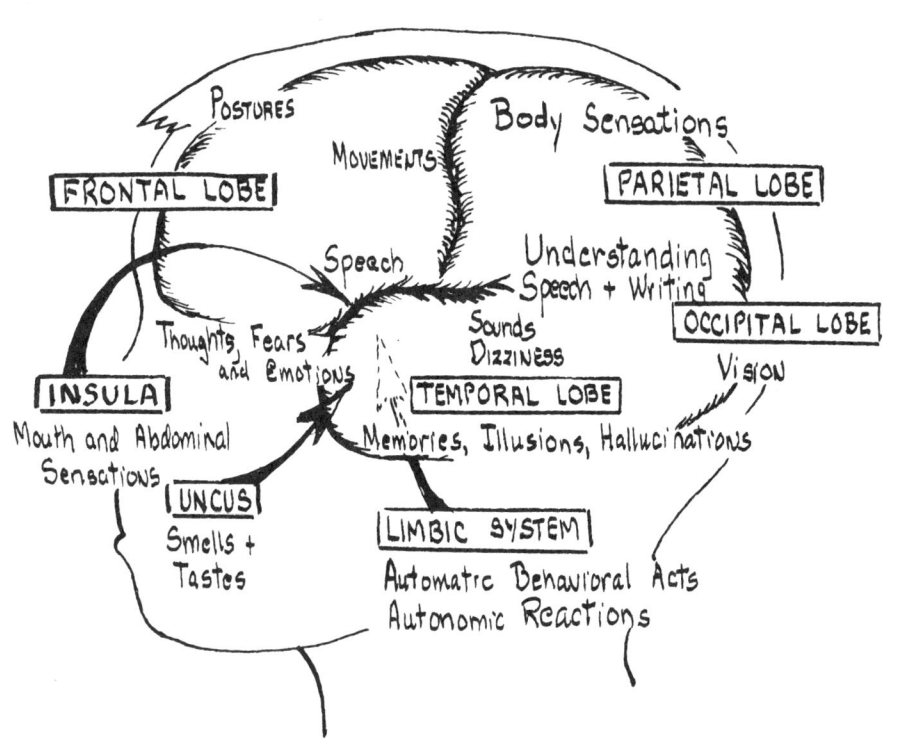

Figure 2.1. Brain areas governing body functions and sensations.

the sensation seems to involve the entire body. Sometimes the sensations are strange and cannot be described. The parietal lobes are often the location of such symptoms. These sensations may be uncomfortable but they are rarely painful.

The patient may note that the early symptoms involve sight. He may complain of blurred vision or actual loss of vision. If the seizure discharge begins in the occipital lobe, he may see blotches, lights, stars, or sparkles. If the discharge is slightly ahead of this area, he may see formed images, illusions, or distortions of what is actually there.

If the discharge begins in the upper portion of the temporal lobe the patient may complain that he hears humming, buzzing, or some familiar sounds, but he rarely hears voices. Another symptom from approximately the same area might be dizziness or a turning sensation.

The patient may complain of unpleasant tastes or smells. Often the discharge is in the medial part of the temporal lobe or the under-surface of the frontal lobe. If the patient's attack begins with a loss of consciousness, dizziness, and confusion, or as a fainting episode, the attack might come from the frontal lobe or occasionally from the temporal lobe.

Early warning symptoms in some patients begin with disturbances in speaking and understanding spoken language. These symptoms usually suggest that the warning comes from the left brain. If the discharge begins in the lower portion of the posterior frontal lobe, the patient mumbles, stammers, or mispronounces words. If it comes from this area or from the anterior temporal lobe, the patient may be unable to speak or at least to speak clearly. If the burst comes from the back portion of the left temporal lobe, the patient may not be able to understand clearly what is being said.

When the temporal lobes are the source of the seizure discharge, warnings involving emotional, behavioral, and thought disturbances are common. The patient may experience strange feelings and emotions. He may have emotional outbursts without any apparent reason, such as screaming, laughing, or crying. He may appear to daydream. He may experience unexplained feelings of loneliness, fear, dread, or anxiety. He may have difficulties in sleeping or else he may be too sleepy. He may have nightmares. Some patients experience only vague, unpleasant sensations that they cannot describe.

The warning-aura may be missed because it was not recognized, was too brief, or was not remembered. A young child or a severely retarded individual may not be able to describe the sensations that he experienced early in the attack.

The Obvious Seizure Attack (or Ictum)

Unlike the warning-aura, the obvious attack is usually quite apparent. The patient is at least confused, if not totally unconscious. Often he displays some movement disturbance, such as tonic stiffening, clonic jerking, single myoclonic jerks, limp akinetic falls, peculiar posturing, or purposeless movements called automatisms. He may just sit and stare without any significant movement. The attack may involve the entire body at once or it may be limited to just a part of the body, such as the face, the hand, or the foot. If the attack begins in one area, it may spread slowly or jump rapidly to involve more of the body.

A great emphasis has been put on whether or not a patient bites his tongue, harms himself, or wets himself. This has been used to determine whether the spell was a seizure or something else. However, this determination is not always helpful. People who fall for other reasons, such as a faint, may harm themselves and bite their tongues. People who faint may occasionally wet themselves. A seizure patient is more apt to wet himself on the way to the bathroom than on the way back. Whether or not the child harms himself or bites his tongue in a seizure depends on what he hits when he falls, and whether or not he chews as part of the seizure. A child who is having a tantrum or hysterical episode usually tries to avoid hurting himself and rarely wets himself.

The degree of the disturbance of consciousness during an attack is important to determine. If the seizure involves part of the body or is limited to only a few symptoms, suggesting that only a part of the brain is involved, the patient may be partially conscious, although confused. If the seizure involves the entire brain in a generalized attack, the patient should be totally unconscious. The patient who remembers what is said and what happens during a generalized attack probably is not having a real seizure. A patient is never completely alert, even when experiencing only a small and very localized seizure attack.

The Recovery Period (Post-Ictum)

When the attack stops, the patient enters into a recovery period. Sometimes this may be very brief, and the patient seems to regain his normal function immediately after the seizure ceases. More often the patient is drowsy to the point of falling into a very deep sleep. If awake, he may have trouble understanding what is being said; he may seem to be confused, agitated, and occasionally jumpy and hyperactive. He may be irritable, complaining of body aches and headaches. He tends to have problems remembering the seizure attack clearly and he may have trouble remembering other facts. He may not speak clearly or choose his words appropriately. He may sit in a daze, performing rather purposeless automatic movements. He may complain of being very tired.

An examination at this time may show some abnormal findings, such as weaknesses in a part of the body (Todd's paralysis), visual disturbances, abnormal reflexes, or language difficulties. Even the brainwave test (EEG) may be quite abnormal at this time. Yet all these symptoms and signs may clear completely within hours to days or occasionally within several weeks at the most. If abnormal findings and functions remain after two to three weeks, they are probably not the aftereffects of the seizure. Beware the patient who remembers too well what happened during a major attack, because such a memory raises suspicions that the attack was not real.

Observers similarly often are vague and confused in their recall and descriptions of the attack. Their panic stretches seconds into minutes and exaggerates some details while overlooking others. Calm assistance in helping the observer give a step-by-step description of what happened may piece together a clearer picture of the attack.

WHAT'S HAPPENING IN THE BRAIN DURING THE SEIZURE

Definition

A seizure is a cluster of symptoms related to an uncontrolled burst of energy originating somewhere in the brain.

Pathoanatomy

The brain cells (neurons) that control brain functions are located in two areas of the brain: 1) on the surface (cortex), or 2) deep in the central portions of the brain (centrencephalic), the brainstem, and the connections to the deeper parts of the surface cortex. These cell collections are the grey matter of the brain. Any brain function is the result of a specific network of these brain cells working together in harmony under the watchful control of other brain cells. Some of these brain cells act as accelerators (or stimulators) and some act as brakes (inhibitors) of the cell networks.

A seizure is the symptomatic result of a sudden and uncontrolled burst of excessive electrical energy involving at least one of these cell networks. Perhaps the controlling cells have lost control. Perhaps the networks, for various reasons, have become disorganized and no longer work in harmony. The problem is not of individual cells gone wild; it is the discharge of energy from a network consisting of many cells that for some reason are no longer working as a team.

Symptomatic Course of the Discharge

Prodromal Build-up During the build-up state, if one occurs, certain areas of the brain begin to lose their efficient functioning as intermittent disturbances of some of the brain cell networks begin to interfere with normal brain activities. The abnormal energies begin to build up with each individual discharge, perhaps lasting longer, becoming stronger, or involving a larger part of the brain.

Warning-Aura When the area of abnormal activity is large enough, lasts long enough, or becomes strong enough, the patient experiences some disturbance of function. What he experiences depends on where in the brain the abnormal discharge occurs. The brain may be able to regain control over this energy before it goes any further. In this case, the patient may experience no further symptoms. However, more commonly the energy builds up further and spreads rapidly to other parts of the brain, like a forest fire out of control.

The Obvious Attack The location of the burst of abnormal energy discharge may be a network of brain cells on the surface (cortex), or some network deep in the central brain areas that connect to the brain surface. If the discharge is localized to some area on the brain surface, the symptoms begin as a specific functional disturbance or a symptom limited to a specific part of the body, such as the hand or the eye. This is a *focal seizure.* The focus tends to spread and enlarge both on the brain and in the body.

The abnormal energy may march across the surface of the brain. In the same fashion, the symptoms, be they a peculiar sensation or jerking, for example, may spread from the beginning focus to adjacent parts of the body. Because of its manner of spread, this is called a *marching seizure.*

A second method of spread is for the focal discharge to spread by deeper nerve pathways from a location on one side of the brain to a related area often on the other side of the brain. Temporal lobe (psychomotor) seizures have this tendency. Within a few years after the development of an abnormal discharge from one temporal lobe, a similar focus may appear in the opposite temporal lobe, like the image of a mirror. This is why the second focus is called a *mirror focus.* Clinically, then, sometimes the seizures seem to begin on one side of the body and sometimes on the other. After several years this mirror focus may become so firmly established that it remains even if the primary focus is removed surgically.

The surface focus may choose a third route for spreading, following nerve pathways to the cell networks located deeper in the middle portions of the brain and brainstem. It then excites these deeper systems to discharges. Since the deeper brain cells tend to relate to activities of the entire brain, such a discharge tends to involve the entire brain at once. The seizure may appear to be a generalized seizure even though the culprit that triggered the seizure was the focal discharge. Therefore, the seizure is considered a focal seizure problem that rapidly becomes generalized. The presence of even a brief warning-aura may be a clue that this focus exists. Often the brainwave test (EEG) reveals a focus in what was clinically thought to be a generalized seizure disorder.

The fourth manner of spread is that seen when the discharge originates in the deeper brainstem cells. The discharge involves all the brain surface at once, or at least it involves critical areas of alertness. This is essentially what happens in the generalized seizure problems. The seizure may present as jerking, stiffening, a single jerk, or a limp drooping, or, if it is limited to the conciousness area, the seizure may present as a brief staring.

The Recovery The brain finally regains control over the erratic discharge only by producing an excess of inhibiting forces. The nervous system is out of balance. Some areas may be receiving too much blood flow and some areas too little. Various chemicals may be present in excess and in other areas there may be a need for vital chemicals. Waste products may have piled up in excess, whereas needed nutritional substances may be deficient. The brain now busies itself in trying to re-establish the balance. The protective inhibiting influences may lead to the slowing of usual brain functions, such as memory, thinking, and alertness. The inhibiting influences may be generalized, although they may be most obvious in the areas where the seizure discharge was most active in the brain. As the storm of abnormal energy calms down, the controlling mechanisms of the brain gradually decrease toward normal functioning. As this occurs, the patient appears to return gradually to his normal state of alertness and function.

CONCLUSION

A seizure is a symptom or a cluster of symptoms related to an abnormal discharge of energy from a network of cells somewhere in the brain. The course of the seizure attack suggests both the origin of the discharge as well as the spread of the abnormal energy burst through the brain; it also suggests the brain's later efforts to inhibit and control the discharge. Although all stages of the seizure may not be present in a seizure attack, it is important that the course of the seizure be recognized, especially early in the onset.

REFERENCES AND SUGGESTED READING

Forster, F. M., and H. E. Booker. 1976. The epilepsies and convulsive disorders. In: A. B. Baker and L. H. Baker (eds.), Clinical Neurology, Vol. 2, 24:1-45. Harper and Row, Hagerstown, Md.

Gowers, W. R. 1881. Epilepsy and Other Chronic Convulsive Diseases: Their Causes, Symptoms and Treatment. Reprinted 1964, Vol. 1, American Academy of Neurology Reprint Series. Dover Publications, Inc., New York. 253 pp.

Lennox, W. G. 1960. Epilepsy and Related Disorders. Little, Brown & Company, Boston. 1168 pp.

Penfield, W., and H. Jasper. 1954. Epilepsy and the Functional Anatomy of the Human Brain. Little, Brown & Company, Boston. 896 pp.

Sands, H., and F. C. Minters. 1977. The Epilepsy Fact Book. F. A. Davis Co., Philadelphia. 116 pp.

3
TYPES OF SEIZURES

Efficient diagnosis and effective management of seizures depend on a clear identification of the attack itself. Accurate classification leads to the selection of the most appropriate diagnostic approaches, to selecting the best medicines and most effective management methods, to an awareness and helping with associated problems, and to an improved understanding of the problems of epilepsy in general.

CLASSIFICATION

For years the major labels applied to seizures included grand mal (greatly bad), petit mal (a little bad), psychomotor, akinetic, and myoclonic. Grand mal attacks include seizures that result in the whole body's stiffening and shaking. Petit mal seizures are attacks of brief stares with little if any movements. Psychomotor seizures are attacks consisting of disturbed emotions, peculiar behaviors, and rather purposeless movements. Akinetic seizures are attacks of falling. Myoclonic seizures present with a body jerk. These terms are vague enough to include many types of attacks and are often loosely applied, resulting in confused understanding and conflicting opinions.

Another approach is to talk of major seizures and minor seizures. In a major seizure there is a major disturbance of movements, usually accompanied by a complete loss of consciousness. The patient falls to the floor. The attack may be either brief or prolonged but it usually does not occur very frequently. Major attacks are so obvious that they are seldom overlooked. By comparison, minor seizures are more subtle and thus are apt to be missed. Movement disturbances are far less prominent. The patient usually does not fall. He may act confused or out of contact but seldom is he completely unconscious. Although minor attacks are shorter in duration, they tend to occur much more frequently than majors. (Another application of the term "minor" is used by some referring to "minor motor seizures," which include the akinetic drop seizures, the myoclonic jerk attacks, and atypical absence stares.) "Minor" and "major" speak only of the severity of the problem; they tell us little more.

Descriptive Onset

Based on modern techniques of observation and study of various seizure types, a better system of classification has been developed in which the emphasis is on noting the earliest symptom or sign of the seizure. The seizure is named for how the attack begins, using descriptive terms, and where in the body it begins, rather than for how bad it is.

The basic brain functions include movements, sensations (including those of touch, sight, sound, smell, and taste), thoughts and memories, emotions, behaviors, speech and language, alertness, and the basic life-support functions of the autonomic nervous system. Each of these functions can be related to a type of seizure and to a specific portion of the brain. The seizure can be described by stating the type of function that was disturbed and what kind of disturbance was noted, as well as whether the disturbance involved a part of the body, half of the body, or the whole body. For example, a seizure might begin as a disturbance of movement, the disturbance being a jerking located in the right arm. Thus we could call this a focal (or localized) clonic (i.e., jerking) motor seizure. Such a description communicates a clearer picture of the attack itself and stimulates considerations of specific concerns regarding causes and other possible problems. It also suggests where in the brain the seizure might have originated. An outline of the various types of seizures, described using the international classification of seizures, is given in Table 3.1.

FOCAL SEIZURE DISORDERS

A focal (or partial) seizure disorder begins in a specific part of the brain rather than beginning all over the brain simultaneously. Consequently, the symptoms begin with the involvement of only a single function, or at most a few functions; they may begin in a small portion of the body. The obvious portions of the attack may be preceded by the warning-aura. This is a clue that the attack is probably a focal seizure disorder, rather than a generalized seizure problem. The patient may be confused during the attack but he is seldom unconscious unless the focus spreads to involve most or all of the brain. Focal seizures have a strong tendency to spread, successively involving larger areas of the brain; consequently, larger areas of the body and an increasing number of functions are involved in the attack as it progresses. When the focus spreads to become large enough, both consciousness and further recall of the seizure events are markedly disturbed. After the attack the patient may experience a temporary loss of a function; this may be a temporary weakness or incoordination of the involved limb, or a speech disturbance, or some such malfunction.

Table 3.1. International classification of seizures

I. Focal or Partial Seizures (seizures beginning locally)
   A. Simple Types (often without a major disturbance of consciousness)
      1. Motor (abnormal movements), including marching-spread
      2. Sensory and special sensory seizures
      3. Disturbances of the autonomic nervous system
      4. Combinations of the above
   B. Complicated Types, usually with a significant disturbance on consciousness (these are often the temporal lobe or psychomotor seizures, or portions of such attacks)
      1. Impaired or disturbed consciousness
      2. Disturbed thinking and memories (cognitive symptoms)
      3. Disturbed emotions or behaviors (affect symptoms)
      4. Psychomotor or psychosensory attacks, including combinations of the above attacks and peculiar sensations (psychosensory) or automatic purposeless movements called automatisms (psychomotor)
      5. Combinations of the above
II. Generalized Seizures (seizures that at the beginning involve the entire body, without focal onset or prominence on one side of the body)
    A. Motor or Movement Disturbances
       1. Too much
          a. Stiffening (tonic) and/or repeated jerking (clonic)
          b. Single jerk or brief cluster of jerks (myoclonic)
       2. Too little
          a. Loss of tone (atonic), of movement (akinetic), or balance (astatic), often with drooping
    B. Staring Spells with Little Movement (Absence)
       1. Typical or simple forms without warning, movement, or aftereffects
       2. Atypical or complicated forms
       3. Mixed forms (absence-akinetic-myoclonic combinations)
III. Unilateral Seizures (involving exclusively or predominantly one side of the body at the onset)
IV. Mixed or Multiple Seizure Disorders (combinations of the above)
V. Neonatal Seizures
   A. Subclinical asymptomatic EEG "seizure bursts"
   B. Subtle or fragmentary neonatal seizures
   C. Multifocal jerking (clonic)
   D. Focal jerking (clonic)
   E. Stiffening (tonic)
   F. Single jerks or small cluster of jerks (myoclonic)
VI. Unclassified seizures (due to the lack of a reliable description or other information about the onset of the attack)

Based on the international classification of epileptic seizures (Gastaut, 1970).

Focal seizures often are misdiagnosed as generalized seizures, even when the warning-aura is present. The focal onset may be overlooked because the warnings were too brief or were not recognized or were too subtle to be observed. Recollection of the key early symptoms may be lost after a major attack. Focal symptoms preceding an attack during sleep are often not noted. The focus may be in a part of the brain that does not present with obvious symptoms to an observer, who thus is not aware of the beginning.

Simple Focal Seizures

Some of the early focal symptoms are fairly simple and straightforward, such as the onset of abnormal stiffening, jerking, or posturing in some part of the body; peculiar and unpleasant (but rarely painful) sensations, sights, sounds, smells, and tastes; dizziness; or a disturbance of the autonomic nervous system's controls over body regulations, such as blood circulation, breathing, the gastrointestinal system, or the genitourinary system. The onset may be a combination of these systems. The patient may be confused, but he is not unconscious unless the seizure spreads to involve a major portion of the brain. Often he can recall early parts of the attack. These simple motor, sensory, and autonomic symptoms are fairly reliable in suggesting where in the brain the abnormal discharge began.

Focal Motor Seizures Focal motor seizures may begin as a tonic stiffening, a clonic jerking, a myoclonic single or brief cluster of jerks, a pause in speech or trouble speaking, a peculiar posturing, a loss in movement, or a break-up of normal coordination. This disturbance of normal movements may begin around the eye, the mouth, in the hand, in the foot, or in some other area of the body. It may then spread to adjacent areas. The initial symptoms may be a deviation of the eyes toward one side opposite the seizure discharge. Motor seizures tend to begin in the part of the brain that falls beneath the band of a pair of earmuffs, with the area controlling the mouth and face being located nearest the ears and the brain area controlling the feet at the top of the head. This area is called the motor strip (see Figure 3.1). Seizures of the left body half usually come from the right brain half and vice versa. Eye deviations can come from either the front or the back of the brain. Speech problems usually come from the left brain half.

Focal Sensory Seizures In focal sensory seizures the initial seizure symptom may be the sensation of tingling, prickling, warmth, coldness, dullness, or heaviness. The patient may be able to localize the sensation to a specific portion of the body or it may appear to be vague and widespread. The sensation may be unpleasant or worrisome but it is rarely painful. These seizures tend to arise from the parietal lobe, which is the part of the brain just behind the motor strip (see Figure 3.2). The sensations that the patient feels are not obvious to an observer and thus are easily missed unless the patient complains about them.

Special Sensory Seizures Some seizures begin with disturbances of sight, hearing, smell, or taste, or as a dizziness. These are the special sensory seizures. With the exception perhaps of the visual seizures, these attacks are not too helpful in telling us which side of the brain is the source of the discharge. Seizures beginning with the distortion of vision or the seeing of

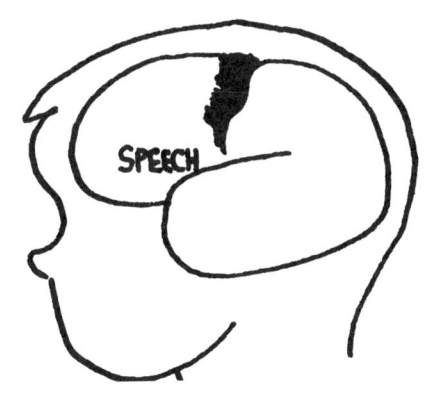

Figure 3.1. The motor strip.

splotches, zig-zags, or spots of light, or of familiar images not actually present, come from the occipital brain lobes, which are located in the very back of the brain (see Figure 3.3). Symptoms like hearing familiar sounds or feeling dizzy (experiencing a turning or spinning sensation) often come from discharges in the temporal lobe. The temporal lobes are located on the lower sides of the brain at about the level of the ears. It is very rare for a person having a seizure to hear voices not present; if this is his main complaint, one must suspect the possibility of an emotional problem. Early symptoms of peculiar and often unpleasant smells and tastes come from beneath the frontal portion of the brain. These sensations rarely relate to anything happening in the patient's environment at the time of the attack.

Autonomic Seizures The autonomic nervous system regulates basic functions and automatic vital functions. Autonomic seizures begin by a disturbance of some of these basic functions. The patient may complain of abdominal cramps or discomfort, of nausea, vomiting, sensations arising in the abdomen and chest, or of peculiar feelings in the throat or mouth.

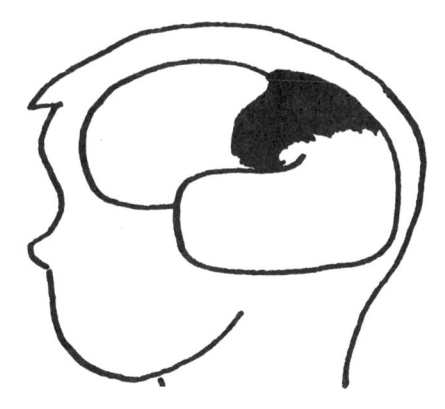

Figure 3.2. The sensory area.

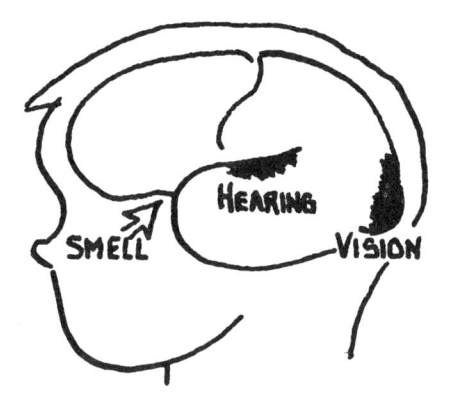

Figure 3.3. Special sensory areas.

Chewing, swallowing, or lip-smacking movements may be seen. The patient may experience irregularities or pauses in breathing or of the heartbeat. His pulse may become fast or slowed; his blood pressure may become high. He may feel hot and appear flushed or he may become pale, cold, and clammy, with shivering and gooseflesh. He may begin to sweat or to have a runny nose, drooling, or an excess of chest secretions. He may complain of peculiar sensations of the bladder or of his sexual organs. His pupils may enlarge. These symptoms often are also seen in other seizure attacks; more often they may be noted in some types of attacks that are not seizures, and with bouts of anxiety and nervousness. With a seizure there is usually a disturbance of consciousness, which is not seen with the other causes of such autonomic symptoms. Autonomic seizures come from deep brain cortex areas away from the outer surface of the brain; they also involve the upper part of the brainstem.

Complicated (or Complex) Focal Seizures

The more complex seizure symptoms usually present as disturbances of thought, memory, emotions, behaviors, and especially consciousness. The patient is apt to be dazed or quite confused, although he is not usually totally unconscious. Despite these symptoms, he may persist in performing complicated acts, such as dressing or undressing. These rather automatic actions are called automatisms. Vague sensations and symptoms of discharges from the autonomic nervous system may be a part of the attacks. Since the seizures tend to come from some part of the temporal lobe or adjacent brain areas (see Figure 3.4), they are often known as temporal lobe seizures. Since they seem to appear as a combination of transient psychological disturbances and the motor automatisms, they have been called psychomotor seizures.

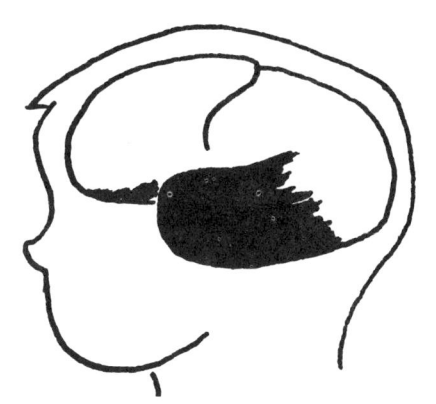

Figure 3.4. The psychomotor area.

Psychomotor Seizures The most typical form of the complex focal or temporal lobe seizure disorders is the psychomotor seizure disorder. Indeed, the other forms of the complex focal seizures may be only fragments of the psychomotor seizure picture. In a full psychomotor seizure the patient appears dazed or quite confused. He may experience disturbing emotions or unexplained and often vague fears. Sometimes he has nightmares. His behavior may change abruptly. He may have peculiar memories or forgetfulness. He may be overcome by persistent strange thoughts. In a variant sometimes known as psychosensory seizures, peculiar but rather vague sensations of the body, complaints of unpleasant smells or tastes, or bothersome dizziness may be prominent. In the more familiar forms of psychomotor seizures, the patient commonly exhibits the movement automatisms. Autonomic nervous system discharges are also commonly noted. When the attack resolves, the patient may seem confused or drowsy, or he may be bothered by a headache.

If the discharge begins in the anterior temporal and lower-underneath portion of the frontal lobe, the automatisms may be a prominent feature. However, attacks beginning with a combination of the automatisms and peculiar posturing followed by a rapid loss of consciousness may come from the back half of the temporal lobe. Discharges from the middle sides and underneath portions of the temporal lobe often begin with a dreamy state, with early disturbances of thought and of emotions noted. Attacks from the upper margins of the temporal lobe or the lowermost portion of the motor strip right above may begin with peculiar sensations, drooling, or movements around the mouth and lips. If dizziness is an early symptom, the upper part of the temporal lobe is the most likely source. If the early symptoms are a combination of facial and mouth movements and prominent autonomic nervous system symptoms, the source of the seizure is most likely to be from the inner surface of the temporal lobe.

In summary, the main symptoms of a psychomotor seizure consist of some combination of distorted consciousness, automatisms, abnormal emotions, disturbed behaviors, peculiar thoughts, erratic memories, autonomic discharges, or abnormal and often rather vague sensations.

Affect (Emotions and Behavior) Disturbances   Some complex focal seizures begin primarily as abrupt emotional upsets, behavioral disturbances, illusions (mistaken sensations), or hallucinations (imagined sensations). These are not stimulated by any current event in the patient's environment. They are of brief duration. The patient may seem confused during and often also after the attack. Specifically, the symptoms may include vague feelings of fear, anxiety, dread, or panic; they may consist of feelings of depression, gloom, worthlessness, despair, rejection, or hopelessness; they may present as feelings of extreme joy or elation. There is no apparent cause for these emotions nor for the associated behavioral outbursts frequently seen, such as sudden bursts of laughter, of non-directed aggression, or of brief bursts of psychotic behavior. Purposeful and planned acts of violence are not seizure behaviors. Affect disturbances, like the cognitive seizures (discussed below), seem to originate from the more primitive brain portions, called the limbic system, as well as from the under-portions of the frontal lobes and the associated anterior and medial portions of the temporal lobes.

Cognitive (Thought and Memory) Disturbances   Some seizures consist primarily of disturbed thoughts or distorted memories, at least in the beginning of the attack. The patient may experience the abrupt onset of a brief period of erratic, faulty, jumbled, or distorted memories. Familiar things may seem strange and strange things may seem familiar. He may experience difficulties in thinking or he may be overwhelmed by recurring thoughts or memories that he cannot put out of his mind. He may feel that his mind is floating outside of his body. During the attack he may appear confused; he may act in a rather erratic and automatic fashion.

Disturbances of Consciousness Only   In some patients the main and perhaps the only symptom is an abrupt but brief loss of consciousness. In the young child the abnormal brain discharge may come from the back part of the temporal lobe; in the older child it is more likely to begin in the anterior temporal or frontal portions of the brain. In some patients the loss of consciousness is followed by the turning of the head and eyes toward the raised arm opposite the seizure focus, whereas in others the head turns to the raised arm before the patient loses consciousness. The sites of the related discharges are in the very front of the brain or the upper-inner surface of the front half of the brain, respectively.

Miscellaneous Focal Seizures of Childhood

In children there are three common types of focal seizures. Some children complain of seeing things that are not really there. The parents note uncontrolled eye movements. The focus of this special sensory seizure is the very back of the brain, the occipital lobe.

A second common focal seizure in children begins with a disturbance of speech. The child appears dazed and confused. Often he may complain of dizziness, headache, numbness, or some other strange feelings of the mouth, the throat, or the abdomen. The observer may note twitching of the mouth or face that rapidly spreads to become a secondarily generalized seizure. This focus commonly comes from the middle to posterior portion of the temporal lobe.

An uncommon type of childhood focal seizure begins in both sides of the front part of the brain. The child rarely experiences any warning-aura. The main problem is one of the episodes of disturbed behavior, some of which may seem almost psychotic. These attacks may come as brief, untriggered episodes or may take on a prolonged waxing and waning nature. The seizures may spread to appear as generalized motor attacks or akinetic drop seizures.

GENERALIZED SEIZURE DISORDERS

The generalized seizure involves the entire body and all body functions from the very beginning of the attack. There rarely is any true warning-aura. If such a warning does occur, perhaps the attack is a focal seizure that becomes secondarily generalized. Indeed, many seizures diagnosed as generalized seizures are really focal seizures that rapidly became generalized, but that did not begin that way. Generalized seizures are thought of as true or primarily generalized seizures and those secondarily generalized seizures that have a focal onset.

In a generalized seizure the patient is markedly out of contact if not totally unconscious. He may experience confusion, drowsiness, and other post-seizure symptoms when the main attack ends, or he may recover as quickly as the seizure began. With the exception of the absence staring seizures, the patient usually falls if he is standing when the seizure occurs. Basically, the major seizure symptoms are: abnormal movements, such as stiffening and jerking; lack of movement; loss of strength and tone, with subsequent falling; or staring episodes. In general, these attacks come from discharges beneath the cortex-surface of the brain and most often from the deeper centers that coordinate the entire brain.

Generalized Motor Seizures

Generalized motor seizures may present with tonic stiffening, clonic repeated jerking, or, more often, with a combination of both. This combination was formerly called grand mal seizures. The attack may begin with an "epileptic cry" as the tightening muscles of the chest suddenly squeeze air out through the tight throat muscles. The patient is completely unconscious from the very beginning. The legs are usually stretched out. The arms may be stretched out or bent up. The back and neck may be arched. The stiffening and jerking interfere with regular breathing and blood circulation; the patient may appear blue or pale or flushed. He may wet himself, bite his tongue or cheeks, vomit, drool, have a bowel movement, or choke and gurgle on excessive chest secretions during the attack. When the attack ends he may be very drowsy, confused, irritable, forgetful, and very sore for a period of time. He may complain of headaches and body aches.

Some young children experience only the tonic stiffening and not the jerking. The arms may be partially bent and raised with the fists clenched. The head is bent forward or backward. The child acts confused, quiet, or irritable for a short time after the attack. This is the tonic seizure of childhood. It is often associated with slowed psychosocial development.

Some individuals immediately enter the clonic jerking phase of the attack without any stiffening portion. This usually is brief but occasionally can go on for hours. These are pure clonic seizures. The typical mixed tonic-clonic attack (true grand mal) is much less common in children than suspected.

Absence Seizures

Absence seizures are staring spells. However, most staring spells that are observed are not seizures, they are boredom. True staring seizures last moments to at most several minutes. They rarely last any longer. Typically there is no warning, no significant movement during the attack, and no aftereffects. The patient is usually briefly "out of contact" but he does not fall. The main component of the attack is a few seconds of blank staring ahead and little more. These attacks may be triggered by deep breathing or less frequently by flashing lights. There are three major groups of staring episodes: the true or simple attacks, the atypical or complicated forms, and some psychomotor seizures that mimic the true absence attacks. These staring attacks were once known as petit mal seizures.

Typical or Simple Absence Seizures In a simple staring attack, the patient stares blankly ahead for from five to twenty seconds. The pupils may enlarge and they may not react to light during the attack. The patient is completely out of contact and unresponsive. The staring and loss of consciousness begin abruptly without any warning and end just as abruptly without any aftereffects. During the attack the patient pauses in his activities; there are no major movements, although the eyelids, and occasionally to a minor degree the face, mouth, or hands, may twitch or flutter at a rate of about three times a second. The patient may appear pale and may sweat during the attack. The patient does not fall, although he may drop items in the middle of the seizure. When the seizure ends, he continues with what he had been doing before the seizure began, often not realizing that he has just had a seizure. As the attack ends, he may blush and his pupils may briefly contract. These attacks may occur up to hundreds of times a day, but they often are more prominent in the morning, after awakening.

Atypical or Complicated Absence Seizures The atypical forms display the basic symptoms of the simple attack plus some variations, such as a brief warning, a brief period of confusion after the spell, or some movements and peculiar behaviors during the attack. The patient may seem confused or partially aware but inattentive during the attack. He is more apt to stare ahead without the rapid eyelid flutter. Some automatisms may be seen, such as licking, chewing, grimacing, yawning, humming, or mumbling. If he was involved in some motor act at the beginning of the attack, he may continue it in an aimless fashion or he may pause in his activities. Some patients may stagger around or walk either forward or backward; some may slump to the ground, whereas others may seem to be thrown backward or forward by the attack. A rare patient may raise and lower his limbs or nod his head in a rapid jerky manner about three times a second or slower. The patient may recall parts of the attack in a confused manner.

These attacks tend to occur less frequently than the typical form. They tend to cluster together; indeed, there may appear to be cycles of clusters of seizures interspaced by relatively seizure-free periods. Strangely, sometimes a painful or sudden stimulus during the attack will stop the seizure. This often leads to a misdiagnosis of emotional seizures.

Psychomotor Absences with Automatisms Some psychomotor seizures can present primarily with staring attacks but these are usually accompanied by automatic movements, such as chewing, yawning, swallowing, playing with clothing, or fumbling with the hands. These attacks may be accompanied by a brief warning-aura and a brief period of confusion after the attack. At times a temporal lobe seizure discharge may fire inward to trigger the generalized atypical absence attack rather than spreading to create more typical psychomotor seizure symptoms.

Drop and Falling Attacks

Two major seizure types that are frequently confused are the akinetic drop seizures and the myoclonic jerk seizures. In an akinetic drop attack, the child suddenly falls limply to the ground without trying to protect himself during his fall with his hands; in the myoclonic jerk attack the patient is hurled forcibly to the ground by the force of the jerk. Akinetic, absence, and myoclonic seizures are occasionally seen in the same patient; this finding used to be called the petit mal triad.

Akinetic, Atonic, and Astatic Drop Attacks The terms akinetic, atonic, and astatic, respectively, mean stopping of normal movements, going limp, and loss of balance. These terms tend to be used interchangeably, with akinetic being the most popular. The patient experiences no warning.

In a full attack he suddenly falls limply to the ground. He may be unconscious so briefly that he may have recovered and be ready to bounce right back up when he hits the ground. If the attack is more prolonged, he may lie there a few seconds or, rarely, minutes before he gets back up. The recovery is usually very rapid, with no confusion. The patient rarely remembers the attack save that he suddenly found himself on the ground. If the seizure is not a full attack, the patient may be seen to nod his head or arm or sag slightly but not to experience a complete fall. He may complain of a momentary weakness of the limb, of momentary stumbling, or of dropping objects. These spells, though brief, may occur many times a day. They are more apt to occur in the mornings or on awakening from sleep.

Myoclonic (Jerk) Seizures A myoclonic seizure consists of one or at most a brief series of jerks involving a part of the body if not the entire body. Not all myoclonic movements are seizures. Some myoclonic jerks can be triggered by sudden sounds, lights, or other external stimuli. The myoclonus may show up as small twitches or ripples in muscles or as violent jerking spasms especially noted in the shoulders or head. The patient may jerk his head downward in a small attack; in a large attack he may be flung violently to the ground, as his entire body is doubled over by the forceful spasm. With the latter attack he is in danger of head injury.

In myoclonic seizures the patient experiences no warning and rarely any aftereffects except the pain of the impact if he falls. He usually does not remember the attack. The seizure is usually very brief, lasting from only fractions of a second to a few seconds at most. There is the tendency for these attacks to occur in clusters rather than to be spaced out. They are more apt to occur in the early morning upon awakening or during the late day when the patient is tired. They seldom occur during sleep. Stress, fatigue, and illness seem to increase the frequency. Clusters of these attacks occasionally can begin to build up in frequency until the patient experiences a tonic-clonic major motor seizure.

In infancy one form of myoclonic spasms may appear that usually is associated with marked slowing down, if not total cessation, of development. The infant may experience warning symptoms or he may give a warning to the parent, such as a color change or an emotional outburst, e.g., a cry or laugh, at the beginning of the attack. The child will suddenly double up, bending his head and body forward, drawing his legs upward, and raising his outstretched arms. Occasionally he may stretch, rather than bend, his legs, or he may do the opposite with the arms. The child may hold this position briefly, with some quivering tremors in the limbs. He is not conscious although he may stare ahead or roll his eyes about. Just as abruptly as the attack begins, it ceases. The child then may be momentarily confused or drowsy but rarely does he fall asleep from the attack. With the end of the spasm the child may cry out or occasionally may sit immobile with a frozen grin on his face. Rarely, the attack may go on to a more typical burst of clonic generalized motor jerking. More often the child experiences a series of one spasm after another, in small clusters, with a brief recovery interval between the spasms.

These attacks come on as fast as lightning. The child seems to fold up suddenly in a flexion spasm, like a jackknife when it is closed. The raised arms, bent legs, and bowed head of the spasm resemble the salaam posture of the Near East. The attack may be limited to head nodding or it may be generalized and extensive in its severity. These characteristics have given rise to many names for these attacks, such as lightning majors, flexion spasms, jackknife seizures, salaam spasms, head-nodding attacks, massive spasms of infancy, etc.

These spasms tend to occur in clusters of rather irregularly spaced attacks, often happening many times a day. Awakening or drowsiness periods seem to accentuate these spells, as does illness, excitement, or strong sensations. As the infant grows older, the spells change; they may be outgrown completely or they may take on the appearance of another type or types of seizures. Unfortunately, the chances are high that the child will be quite slowed in intellectual and perhaps motor development.

The typical attack as described usually lasts around a second for each spasm. A related form is a very rapid sudden total body flexion that lasts but a fraction of a second. These attacks often are triggered by external sensations, such as sound or touch. They occur irregularly, depending somewhat on the frequency of the triggering sensations. Because the overall outlook is so poor for an infant who develops myoclonic spasms, an intensified search for a possible treatable cause is begun as soon as the diagnosis is even suspected.

UNILATERAL SEIZURE DISORDER

Some seizures seem to originate predominately, if not exclusively, from one-half of the body, and thus the opposite half of the brain. A specific focus within the affected brain may not be apparent, although further studies frequently may reveal the subtle focal discharge.

One severe form of unilateral seizures is the Lennox Gastaut syndrome. The child experiences a progressive and usually pharmacologically uncontrollable unilateral seizure disorder. The attacks consist of focal to rapidly generalizing motor seizures of various types. Atypical absence staring attacks and psychomotor seizures may also be seen. These attacks tend to occur in clusters and the clusters most often happen at night. As the seizures continue, the child's overall function tends to deteriorate. By adolescence the child may be handicapped by the loss of intelligence and function although the seizures may be outgrown.

MULTIFOCAL — MIXED — SEIZURE DISORDERS

In some patients a careful history and good observation will indicate that they are experiencing more than one or two types of seizures. There may be a combination of focal and generalized attacks, including a mixture of focal motor, myoclonic jerk, atypical absence staring, psychomotor, tonic stiffening, and clonic jerking attacks. The generalized attacks may actually be spread from focal beginnings. The existence of the multiple types of seizures suggest that there are multiple areas of the brain that are discharging independently. This situation can be verified by further studies. Such a condition is often labeled a mixed seizure disorder, with the principal seizure types then listed.

NEONATAL (NEWBORN) SEIZURES

Neonatal seizures are often brief, atypical, and overlooked. In a decreasing order of frequency, the most common type of attack is that of a subtle or fragmentary seizure rather than a more typical episode. More obvious seizure attacks may occur, including jerking movements or tremors in many areas of the body, or, occasionally, just in one area, stiffening attacks, and occasionally even sudden jerks of the body. The seizure is a worrisome signal of the intensity of an insult to the newborn infant; it neither localizes the problem in the brain nor hints at what the cause might be. Due to the immature development of the brain, the location of the seizure on the body does not necessarily relate to any specific part of the brain.

Initial seizures may be overlooked. Neonatal seizures tend to be small, brief, and often limited to the face or hand. Small, recurring episodes may present as brief pauses in activities, such as eating, breathing, or stretching, as brief staring spells, as bursts of eye rolling or jerking of the eyes (nystagmus), as twitching or winking of the face, as chewing, sucking, or other mouthing movements, or as small twitches or tremors of the limbs. These few seconds of abnormal activities may be the entire seizure, and they are the more typical forms of seizures in the neonate. Often they are best picked up by watching the infant's face directly while keeping the limbs in view also. More familiar seizure symptoms, such as stiffening, jerking, loss of consciousness, or drowsiness after an attack, are less frequently seen. The seizures tend to be very short although fairly frequent. They usually are not long enough to interfere with breathing. It is most desirable to note and to respond to seizures early, for if these early signals of the underlying brain irritation are overlooked until the basic problem becomes worse, the later appearance of more typical seizures may lead to a poorer outlook.

UNCLASSIFIED SEIZURE DISORDERS

After the neonate period, seizures can and should be classified specifically, provided enough information is available about the way the attack began. Sometimes this information is lacking. Sometimes the appearance of the seizure seems to change from one attack to the next, so that there is not any typical pattern. Sometimes the cause, be it a fever, a flashing light, or a blow to the head, is more apparent than the seizure response. Sometimes spells are unclassified because they neither resemble a seizure nor are actually seizures. When one is not sure of the classification, it is far more honest to state that the seizure is an unclassified seizure disorder... at least until enough information becomes available to classify the attacks more specifically. The label "unclassified seizure disorder" must be considered a temporary term and an obligation exists to replace it with a more accurately documented term by careful observation and evaluation.

APPLIED CLASSIFICATION

Classifying the seizure is not hard if the observer notes the beginning features. If the patient is a newborn child, the classification already is made. Beyond the newborn period, good observation is needed. If there is not enough dependable information about the seizure, it is best to use the term "unclassified" and to realize that this implies an obligation to classify the attacks more specifically through further observation and studies.

The primary classification questions are *where* and *how* the seizure began. The seizure either begins in a part of the body, one side of the body, or all over the body at the onset. Thus the terms focal, unilateral, or generalized can be applied, respectively. The initial symptoms may be disturbance of movement, of sensation or special sensations, of thought, of emotion, of behavior, of alertness and consciousness, or of the autonomic life-support system. The terms motor, sensory, special sensory, psychomotor, affect (emotions), cognitive (thoughts), absence stares, or autonomic may be applied as indicated.

Then the particular function disturbance must be considered. A motor functional disturbance may be jerking (clonic), stiffening (tonic), a single spasmodic jerk (myoclonic), a drop (akinetic), a peculiar posture, or an automatism, for example. Describing the type of disturbance of function can give a further picture of the seizure.

The final consideration in describing the seizure is whether there was any stimulus or sensation that might have caused the seizure to occur. This topic is discussed in the next chapter.

REFERENCES AND SUGGESTED READING

General Discussions

Bruya, M. A., and R. H. Bolin. 1976. Epilepsy: A controllable disease. Classification and diagnosis of seizures. Am. J. Nurs. 76:388-397.

Castle, G. F., and L. S. Fishmann. 1973. Seizures. Pediatr. Clin. North Am. 20: 819-835.

Fois, A. 1963. Clinical Electroencephalography in Epilepsy and Related Conditions in Children. Charles C Thomas, Springfield, Illinois. 268 pp.

Forster, F. M., and L. H. Booker. 1976. The epilepsies and convulsive disorders. In: A. B. Baker and L. H. Baker (eds.), Clinical Neurology, Vol. 2, 24:1-45. Harper and Row Publishers, Hagerstown, Maryland.

Gomez, M. R., and D. W. Klass. 1972. Seizures and other paroxysmal disorders in infants and children. Current Problems in Pediatrics, Vol. 2, Nos. 6 and 7. Year Book Medical Publishers, Inc., Chicago. 38 pp.

Gowers, W. R. 1881. Epilepsy and Other Chronic Convulsive Diseases: Their Causes, Symptoms and Treatment. Reprinted 1964. Vol. 1, American Academy of Neurology Reprints. Dover Publications, Inc., New York. 253 pp.

Jeras, J., and I. Tivadar. 1973. Epilepsies in Children. The University Press of New England, Hanover, N. H. 143 pp.

Lennox, W. G. 1960. Epilepsy and Related Disorders. Little, Brown & Company, Boston. 1168 pp.

Livingston, S. 1972. Comprehensive Management of Epilepsy in Infancy, Childhood and Adolescence. Charles C Thomas, Springfield, Illinois, 657 pp.

Magnus, O., and A. M. Lorentz de Haas (eds.). 1974. The Epilepsies. In: P. J. Vincken and G. W. Bruyn (eds.), Handbook of Clinical Neurology, Vol. 15. North Holland Publishing Co., Amsterdam, and American Elsevier Publishing Co., New York. 860 pp.

Singer, H. S., and J. M. Freeman. 1975. Seizures in adolescents. Med. Clin. North Am. 59:1461-1472.

Solomon, G. E., and F. Plum. 1976. Clinical Management of Seizures. W. B. Saunders Company, Philadelphia. 152 pp.

Classification

Gastaut, H. 1969. Clinical and electroencephalographic classification of epileptic seizures. Epilepsia 10 (Suppl.):2-13.

Gastaut, H. 1969. Classification of the epilepsies. Proposal for an international classification. Epilepsia 10 (Suppl.):14-21.

Masland, R. L. 1969. Comments on the classification of epilepsy. Epilepsia 10 (Suppl.):22-27.

Specific Seizure Types

Charlton, M. H. 1975. Myoclonic Seizures. Roche Medical Monograph Series — Excerpta Medica. Hoffman-LaRoche, Inc., Nutley, New Jersey. 167 pp.

Dreifuss, F. E. 1975. The differential diagnosis of partial seizures with complex symptomatology. In: J. K. Penry and D. D. Daly (eds.), Advances in Neurology, Vol. 11, Chap. 9. Raven Press, New York.

Gomez, M. 1969. Prenatal and neonatal seizure disorders. Postgrad. Med. 46: 71-77.

Jeavons, P. M. 1977. Nosological problems of myoclonic epilepsies in childhood and adolescence. Dev. Med. Child Neurol. 19:3-8.
Jeavons, P. M., and B. D. Bower. 1964. Infantile Spasms. Clinics in Developmental Medicine, No. 15. Wm. Heinemann Medical Books Ltd., London. 82 pp.
Livingston, S., and I. Pruce. 1978. Petit mal epilepsy. Family Physician 17:1-7-114.
Lombroso, C. T. 1974. Seizures in the newborn period. In: O. Magnus and A. M. Lorentz de Haas (eds.), The Epilepsies (Vol. 15 of P. J. Vincken and G. W. Bruyn (eds.), Handbook of Clinical Neurology), Chap. 9:189-218. North Holland Publishing Co., Amsterdam, and American Elsevier Publishing Co., Inc., New York.
Menkes, J. H. 1976. Diagnosis and treatment of minor motor seizures. Pediatr. Clin. North Am. 23:435-442.
Ounsted, C., J. Lindsay, and R. Norman. 1966. Biological Factors in Temporal Lobe Epilepsy. Clinics of Developmental Medicine, No. 22. Wm. Heinemann Medical Books Ltd., London, 135 pp.
Werner, S. S., J. E. Stockard, and R. G. Bickford. 1977. Atlas of Neonatal Electroencephalography. Raven Press, New York. 211 pp.

4
CAUSES OF SEIZURES

A seizure is not a disease, it is only a symptom of something interfering with normal brain function. Although the tendency to develop seizures may be inherited, more often the seizure is due either to an ongoing insult or to the scars left from a previous insult to the brain. The primary purpose of the seizure evaluation is to ensure that there is no ongoing brain insult that could prove to be damaging or even fatal. The information gained from a good evaluation can also be used to counsel the patient and his family about the impact of the seizure problem on the patient's life and on his relatives and offspring.

A scientist looks at a seizure as being the result of an erratic burst of energy from a cluster of interconnected nerve cells located somewhere in the brain. The system may be unrestrained, damaged, or disorganized; it may be immature, overly sensitized, or excessively irritated. Sometimes a cluster of cells seems to work independently from the rest of the brain. Any of these conditions can result in seizures and other symptoms.

Seizures can be considered as either an inherited tendency or an acquired problem. Sometimes both factors seem to be causes in the same patient. Often a cause is not apparent despite an intensive evaluation. This is commonly called an idiopathic seizure disorder, meaning that the cause is not known. Many, but not all, of the idiopathic seizures probably are acquired disturbances.

INHERITED SEIZURE PROBLEMS

Within the limits of present genetic knowledge, it is difficult to develop a clear picture of the chances of inheriting or passing on a seizure tendency. The family history is often obscured by vague descriptions, incorrect labels, inadequate medical histories, and hidden or denied epileptic relatives. Obviously, those seizures related to some brain insult are most likely not going to be inherited.

Some seizure *tendencies* may be inherited, although the abnormality may only appear on a brainwave tracing and not as a clinical symptom. It is not yet known why some individuals have the seizures and some only the abnormal brainwave patterns and no attacks. The two common patterns of inheritance of a seizure tendency are by an autosomal dominant pattern and by a sex-linked pattern. With either pattern each child stands a fifty-fifty chance of inheriting the tendency. With a sex-linked pattern, the male who inherits the tendency is most likely to have the seizures, whereas the female who inherits the trait probably will not have the seizure problem. Both can pass it on. With autosomal dominant inheritance, either sex can inherit the tendency and pass it on and either sex can have the seizures. There probably are more ways of inheriting a seizure disorder than the two given above, but these others have not been clearly defined.

Some types of seizures are more apt to be inherited. Febrile seizures in young children, seizures triggered by flashing lights, and simple absence attacks have a strong tendency toward being inherited. With the absence seizures, each child has a 50% chance of inheriting the brainwave abnormality but only a 25% chance of having the seizures. Obviously, with any kind of seizure, if the parent and child, two siblings, or multiple relatives have the same type of seizure and there is no known common cause, the chances are strong that this may be an inherited seizure disorder. If one identical twin develops a seizure problem without any apparent cause, the other probably will develop at least the EEG abnormality, if not the seizures.

Inherited seizures tend to appear in early childhood and usually before mid-adolescence. As the child grows from his preschool years toward adolescence and young adulthood without a seizure occurring the likelihood of his having inherited a seizure disorder decreases.

MIXED SEIZURE CAUSES

Some patients have a positive family history suggesting a hereditary seizure tendency and a medical history and examination that indicate a probable insult to the brain that also could have caused the seizure problem. The patient may have inherited the seizure tendency, which was brought out by the insult. For example, the patient may inherit a tendency to develop temporal lobe seizures. The temporal lobe structures thus may be more vulnerable to the insults of birth, of high fevers, or of metabolic upset in early life. Consequently, the child develops a temporal lobe seizure problem although the insult may not seem severe.

IDIOPATHIC AND ACQUIRED SEIZURE DISORDERS

There are numerous causes for seizures. A seizure disorder may be inherited as a tendency or it may be the result of a present or prior insult to the brain, interfering with normal brain function or leading to brain damage. Types of insults include disturbances of body metabolism, chemical imbalances, drug reactions, poison ingestion, breathing problems, disturbances of blood circulation to the brain, fever, infections, immunization reactions, allergic and immune reactions, trauma, tumors, malformations, abnormalities of blood vessels (including bleeding or blockage), degenerative disorders, or sensory hypersensitivity. This is by no means a complete list. Many times a cause is not found. However, a careful consideration of four factors may help to indicate the most likely causes to investigate, namely: 1) the type of seizure, 2) the circumstances surrounding the attack, 3) the age of the patient when the seizure began, and 4) the course of the seizure pattern since the onset.

THE TYPES OF SEIZURES

Generalized Seizures

Insults that tend to affect the entire brain diffusely rather than concentrating in any one area tend to cause generalized seizures. It is true that generalized seizures are more likely to be inherited than are focal or multifocal seizures; however, the majority of the generalized seizures, with the exception possibly of the simple absence attacks, are acquired problems.

The major known causes of a generalized seizure disorder include: 1) infections or inflammations of the brain, the brain coverings, or the blood vessels of the brain; 2) chemical upsets and inborn metabolic errors; 3) poison ingestions or drug reactions; 4) degenerative disorders of the nervous system; or 5) allergic and immune reactions following viral infections and immunizations.

Most generalized seizures do not have an apparent cause. However, those seizures associated with a significant disturbance in learning, significant abnormalities on the neurologic exam, or significantly abnormal findings on the brainwave test are most likely acquired disorders. Atypical absence, akinetic, myoclonic, and generalized tonic seizures are usually acquired seizure disorders.

Multifocal Seizures

A diffuse insult of the nervous system may result in multifocal seizures. Often the source of the insult is outside the nervous system, as with a problem in breathing, blood circulation, or body chemistry and metabolism. Metastatic tumors, systemic malformations, and inflammations of the blood vessels also can cause multifocal seizure problems. In all cases the brain is secondarily affected. Usually the intelligence is lower, the examination (including a general physical) is significantly abnormal, and the EEG shows the multiple seizure foci.

Focal Seizures

Problems causing an irritation or scarring of specific areas of the brain result in focal seizures. Occasionally there may be a family history of similar seizures, but focal seizures are essentially considered acquired disorders. The seizure may be due to an active irritation or it may result from scars left by a previous insult damaging a part of the brain. Such insults as blood vessel abnormalities (hemorrhages and blocks), masses (tumors, blood clots, cysts, or abscesses), malformations of the brain or blood vessels, and trauma must be considered. Often the learning processes, the neurologic examination, and the EEG are abnormal, with a tendency toward localizing features.

Sometimes a focal seizure is triggered by one of the disturbances usually associated with generalized seizure disorders. When an insult such as low blood sugar or calcium levels, an infection, lack of oxygen, or a disturbance of blood flow triggers a focal convulsion, one must consider that a focal defect may already have been present and was triggered by the added insult. Because of the peculiar structure of the inner part of the temporal lobe, metabolic deficiencies, lack of oxygen, or brain swelling may produce focal damage to this area, resulting in later psychomotor convulsions.

TIMING AND CIRCUMSTANCES OF THE SEIZURE PROBLEM

A good description of the timing of and circumstances surrounding the seizure attack may point out an obvious cause. Some seizures occur only at the time of an insult to the brain: e.g., head trauma; a low blood sugar, calcium, or oxygen over or under supply; a disturbance in the blood flow to the brain; or an extremely high fever. These should be called secondary seizures because they are secondary to whatever the primary problem is. However, if the patient has a seizure tendency already present, the insult may only activate the tendency. The insult also can cause brain damage and later seizures. These should be considered primary seizure disorders. Primary seizures, unlike secondary seizures, tend to recur under other circumstances and usually can be demonstrated by a significantly abnormal brainwave tracing. Both problems respond to therapy, although a secondary seizure disorder may not need to be treated if the insult can be prevented from happening again.

Secondary Seizures

Infections and Fevers If the patient has a meningitis, an encephalitis, or an inflammation of the blood vessels of the brain, he may experience a secondary seizure. It is not apt to occur again in the future unless the infection leaves a scar.

Sometimes a systemic infection that does not involve the brain directly may result in high fever that triggers a convulsion. Infants and young children are especially prone to this reaction because of the immaturity of their brains. In this group, the seizure is called a "febrile seizure." In older individuals it usually takes an extremely high fever to cause a seizure.

Typically, a simple febrile seizure is a problem seen in children between the ages of 6 months and 3 to 5 years. The child has a seizure triggered by a fever that is at least 103°. The seizure usually lasts only 5 to 10 minutes and not more than 20 minutes; it usually is generalized and it rarely recurs. If the attack does recur, it seldom recurs more than once. There may be a family history of a similar problem. The medical history is negative for any birth or other insults to the brain. The child's development is fairly normal. The neurologic examination, an examination of the cerebrospinal fluid, and the EEG obtained several weeks later are all essentially normal. Whether a simple febrile seizure needs to be treated beyond intensified fever control is still being debated.

The atypical or complicated febrile seizure does not meet the criteria of the simple febrile attack. The attack may occur outside of the age ranges given above, it may occur with a low fever, and it may be prolonged, focal, or recurrent. The previous history, the development, the examination, and the EEG may be abnormal. The greater the number of deviations from the simple picture, the greater are the chances of this being a primary seizure tendency activated by a fever. This is especially true if the EEG is definitely abnormal. The patient is usually given regular anticonvulsant therapy.

Food Some seizures tend to occur early in the morning or when a meal is missed or delayed. This suggests that the problem may be related to low blood sugar and inadequate reserves. Some seizures seem to relate to meals, and especially to the eating of certain foods. This suggests the problem may be a metabolic disorder. The aggravating foods may trigger an abnormal fall in blood sugar or a rise in blood ammonia.

Sleep Irregularities In a few individuals, loss of sleep, and, in other individuals, an excess of sleep may be the only cause of a seizure. Drowsiness also may tend to bring out seizures in general. An EEG may help delineate the problem. Certainly the history suggests that a change in the sleeping patterns should be part of the therapy.

Menstrual Periods and Pregnancies Some girls find that their seizures are aggravated by, if not limited to, the time of or before their menstrual period. Some women find that their seizures occur during pregnancies, even when their blood pressure is normal. Moderate fluid and salt restriction and the use of Diamox during the seizure-prone period, in addition to ongoing anticonvulsant therapy, may help control these attacks.

Reflex Sensory Seizures

There are certain individuals who will have a convulsion whenever they are exposed to a specific sensory stimulus. The triggering sensation may be: a flickering or shimmering light; a specific pattern or color; a certain tone, pitch, melody, or rhythm; a touch or tap on a specific area on the body; or even the act or thought of a movement. Common situations triggering such seizures include a faulty TV picture, reflected light from a window or a body of water, sunlight flickering through a row of trees or onto a windshield, sitting too close to or too far to the side of a movie screen, or listening to certain types of music. The basic ingredients seem to be a rhythmic sensory stimulation pattern and a prolonged or intensified exposure.

These sensations are registered in brain centers that may be immature or overly sensitive and consequently over-reactive. The initial symptoms may be a feeling of light-headedness or dizziness, a vague discomfort, or a dull headache. The patient may act confused, stare, blink, or exhibit myoclonic jerks and twitches of the eyelids, face, head, and even the shoulders. If the stimulus is continued, a major seizure may occur.

This tendency may be inherited. It may even be pleasurable; often the patients may be seen trying to recreate the triggering stimulus. They may seek out and gaze at bright lights, waving their fingers before their eyes, or they may purposefully purchase specific records. A good history often uncovers the stimulating circumstance, indicating the need for sensory stimulation as part of the brainwave testing, and opens the door to alternate methods of treatment (see Chapter 11).

AGE OF ONSET OF THE SEIZURE PROBLEM

There are certain ages when seizures are more apt to occur, certain seizures that are apt to begin at specific ages, and certain types of problems that are more apt to be present at specific age periods. The age of the true onset of the seizure disorder suggests possible causes. Sometimes the supposed age of onset is not the real onset, since after the diagnosis has been confirmed the parents may recall prior peculiar behaviors that were probably also seizures.

The peak ages of seizure occurrence are in the newborn period, in late infancy, and in early adolescence and pre-adolescence (from about 9 to 15 years of age). Seizures may occur before birth, but this is rare. Neonatal seizures are most commonly subtle fragmentary reactions to active brain irritations. Seizures before 6 months of age are uncommon and usually indicate an active brain insult or an anatomic defect. In later infancy, seizures are more common. They tend to become rapidly generalized even when the onset is focal. At this age myoclonic spasms and febrile seizures may occur. During the preschool years akinetic attacks may develop, whereas absence attacks become noted more often in the early school years. Temporal lobe and other focal seizures become prominent problems in the pre-teen and adolescent years. In the second decade and thereafter, focal seizure disor-

Table 4.1. Peak periods for various causes of seizures

	Newborn	Infant	Child	Teen	Adult	Elderly
Trauma	XXXXX	XXXXXXXXXXXXXXXXXXXXX
Malformation	XXXXXXXXXX
Infection	XXXXXXXXXX
Birth insult	XXXXXXXXXXXXXX
Metabolic problem	XXXXXXXXXXXXXX
Drugs, poisons, etc.	XXXXX	XXXX	XXXXXXXX		XXXXX
Vascular problems	XXXXXXXXXXXXXXXXXXX		XXXXXXX
Degenerations		XXXXXXXX
Immunizations	XXXXXXX
Fever	XXXXXXX
Reflex sensitivity	XXXXXXXXX
Inherited	XXXXXXXXXX
Idiopathic		XXXXXXXX
Tumor		XXXXXXXXXXXXXXX

ders become more prominent and more alarming because of the increased risks that the cause may be a brain tumor. The peak periods for various causes of seizures are given in Table 4.1.

Seizures caused by infections, fevers, malformations, and immunizations usually begin during the first five years of life; those due to birth insults, inborn metabolic errors, and degenerative disorders usually begin in the first ten years of life and often in the first five years. Inherited seizure problems tend to appear by early adolescence, whereas idiopathic seizure problems often begin before mid-adolescence. Primary brain tumors are an increasing cause of seizures in the older child, the adolescent, and especially the adult, although the immature 'blastic' tumors and leukemias may spread to the brain in younger children. Trauma, drugs, poisons, and vascular disturbances can result in seizures at any age.

THE COURSE OF THE SEIZURE DISORDER

A seizure may present as an acute problem or as a chronic disturbance. If it is a chronic problem, the pattern may be stable and unchanging or it may be a changing pattern. Changing seizure patterns are danger signals.

Acute Seizures

An acute and active insult can generate a seizure reaction. The insult may be an infection, a poison, or a drug reaction, a vascular problem, a metabolic disturbance, a mass in the head, or trauma. The seizure may be the first attack with many to follow. The evaluator searches for acute insults. Often the search includes screens for disturbances in the body chemistry, for inborn metabolic errors, and for poisons and drugs, as well as an examination of the cerebrospinal fluid, in addition to the basic diagnostic procedures.

Chronic Seizures

The approach to a chronic seizure disorder is somewhat different. With the passage of time, the chances that the cause is an infection, a hemorrhage, a poison, a drug reaction, trauma, or a fast-growing tumor diminishes, although masses, malformations, and scars from previous insults still are to be considered. A changing seizure pattern is of concern because it implies an ongoing problem. Changes may be due to alterations in the therapy, or, in the case of a young child, the change may relate to the maturation of the brain. The concerns with a changing seizure picture are that the cause might be a slow-growing mass, a vascular malformation, a chronic infection, an inherited metabolic disturbance, or a degenerative disorder of the brain. An intensive evaluation or re-evaluation is necessary so that nothing is overlooked that might be treated and possibly cured.

CONCLUSIONS

Rather than a frantic attempt to exclude any and all of the numerous causes of seizures, a thoughtful review of the pertinent characteristics of the seizure problem may indicate the most likely causes of the convulsions. The type of seizure, the age of onset, the circumstances around the attacks, and the course of the seizure problem may spotlight or focus on the areas of concern, and indicate whether the seizure problem is an acquired disturbance or an inherited tendency. Seizures of an acute onset, of a changing pattern, or of a focal or multifocal type are particularly worrisome, requiring most intensive evaluations and closer follow-up care.

REFERENCES AND SUGGESTED READING

General

Alter, M., and W. A. Hauser. 1973. The Epidemiology of Epilepsy: A Workshop. NINDS Monograph No. 14. DHEW Publication No. (NIH) 73-390. U.S. Government Printing Office, Washington, D.C. 167 pp.

Bergamini, L., B. Bergamasco, P. Benna, and M. Gilli. 1977. Acquired etiological factors in 1,785 epileptic subjects: clinical-anamnestic research. Epilepsia 18:437-444.

Epilepsy Foundation of America. 1975. Basic Statistics on the Epilepsies. F. A. Davis Company, Philadelphia. 155 pp.

Forster, F. M., and L. H. Booker. 1976. The epilepsies and convulsive disorders. In: A. B. Baker and L. H. Baker (eds.), Clinical Neurology, Vol. 2, 24:1. Harper and Row Publishers, Hagerstown, Maryland.

Gomez, M. R., and D. W. Klass. 1972. Seizures and other paroxysmal disorders in infants and children. Current Problems in Pediatrics, Vol. 2, Nos. 6 and 7. Year Book Medical Publishers, Inc., Chicago, 38 pages each.

Lennox, W. G. 1960. Epilepsy and Related Disorders. Little, Brown & Company, Boston. 1168 pp.

Livingston, S. 1956. Etiologic factors in adult convulsions. An analysis of 689 patients whose attacks began after twenty years of age. New Engl. J. Med. 254:1211-1216.

Livingston, S. 1972. Comprehensive Management of Epilepsy in Infancy, Childhood and Adolescence. Charles C Thomas, Springfield, Illinois. 657 pp.

Solomon, G. E., and F. Plum. 1976. Clinical Management of Seizures. W. B. Saunders Company, Philadelphia. 152 pp.

Genetic Studies

Doose, H., H. Gerken, T. Horstmann, and E. Volzke. 1973. Genetic factors in spike-wave absence. Epilepsia 14:57-76.

Eisner, V., L. L. Pauli, and S. Livingston. 1959. Hereditary aspects of epilepsy. Bull. Johns Hopkins Hosp. 105:245-271.

Fleiszar, K. A., W. L. Daniel, and P. B. Imrey. 1978. Genetic study of infantile spasms with hypsarrhythmia. Epilepsia 18:55-62.

Lindsay, M. M. M. 1971. Genetics and epilepsy: A model from critical path analysis. Epilepsia 12:47-54.

Metrakos, J. D., and K. Metrakos. 1966. Childhood epilepsy of subcortical ("centrencephalic") origin. Clin. Ped. 5:536-542.

Neonatal Seizures

Gomez, M. 1969. Prenatal and neonatal seizure disorders. Postgrad. Med. 46:71 77.

Febrile Seizures

Chevrie, J. J., and J. Aicardi. 1975. Duration and lateralization of febrile convulsions. Etiologic factors. Epilepsia 16:781-790.

Nelson, K. B., and J. H. Ellenberg. 1976. Predictors of epilepsy in children who have experienced febrile seizures. New Engl. J. Med. 295:1029-1033.

Pollack, M. A. 1978. Continuous phenobarbital treatment after a "simple febrile convulsion." Am. J. Dis. Child. 132:87-89.

Shaw, R. F., J. C. Gall, Jr., and S. H. Schuman. 1972. Febrile convulsions as a problem in waiting times. Epilepsia 12:305-311.

Taylor, D. C., and C. Ounsted. 1971. Biological mechanisms influencing the outcome of seizures in response to fever. Epilepsia 12:33-46.

Wolfe, S. M. 1977. Effectiveness of daily phenobarbital in the prevention of febrile seizure recurrences in "simple" febrile convulsions and "epilepsy triggered by fever." Epilepsia 18:95-99.

Reflex Seizures

Forster, F. M. 1972. The classification and conditioning treatment of the reflex epilepsies. Int. J. Neurol. 9:73-86.

Green, J. B. 1971. Reflex epilepsy. Electroencephalographic and evoked potential studies of sensory precipitated seizures. Epilepsia 12:225-234.

Jeavons, P. M., and G. F. A. Harding. 1975. Photosensitive Epilepsy. Clinics in Developmental Medicine, No. 56. Wm. Heinemann Medical Books Ltd., London, and J. B. Lippincott Company, Philadelphia. 121 pp.

Temporal Lobe Epilepsy

Falconer, M. A. 1971. Genetic and related aetiological factors in temporal lobe epilepsy. A review. Epilepsia 12:13-32.

Heijbel, J., S. Blom, and M. Rasmuson. 1975. Benign epilepsy of childhood with centro-temporal EEG study: A genetic study. Epilepsia 16:285-294.

Ounsted, C., J. Lindsay, and R. Normal. 1966. Biologic Factors in Temporal Lobe Epilepsy. Clinics of Developmental Medicine, No. 22. Wm. Heinemann Medical Books Ltd., London. 135 pp.

5
EXAMINING THE PATIENT

Seizures are human problems, not laboratory phenomena. Therefore, a good history and examination are necessary in order to select the appropriate laboratory tests, to understand the test results, to choose the best methods of management of the attacks and related problems, and to counsel the patient and his family.

HISTORY

The major goals of the history taking are: 1) to obtain a good understanding of the characteristics of the seizures, 2) to identify any possible causes, 3) to become aware of any other problems needing help, and 4) to determine the effects of previous treatment.

Characterizing the Seizure

The main need is to characterize the seizure completely, in an orderly, step-by-step fashion. The description should be able to recreate a mental picture of the attack in the mind of anyone reviewing the evaluation. Such a picture covers not only the blow-by-blow description of the seizure itself, but also the time, the frequency, and the duration of each attack, the circumstances in which the attack occurred, and the age of onset for each seizure type. The course of the seizure also is important.

Drug History

A full review of the effects of present and previous medications (and of any other management approaches) should be made. The main questions for each medication are: 1) What was it? 2) Did it help? or 3) Did it have any bad effects?

Identifying the name of the medication, the strength and form (liquid, syrup, capsule, or tablet), and the frequency of administration per day is important, especially for presently used drugs; it is also desirable for previously used medicines. The patient and his family may be unsure of the names and strengths of the drugs. A plasticized display board or a colored chart containing the anticonvulsant drugs, as well as other commonly used medications (stimulants, tranquilizer, etc.) may be a helpful aid in obtaining proper identification. The cause for reactions or non-response to the drug may be found by calculating the total daily dosage as compared to the child's weight. By comparing the calculated dosage to usual dosage ranges it may be discovered that the dosage was too strong or too weak. It may also be found that the manner of giving the medication or the form used was inappropriate.

The effects, both good and bad, of all previous and present medications should be noted, including both anticonvulsants and other drugs used. If the drug was helpful, exactly how did it help, and which seizures or behaviors seemed to respond favorably? If the drug had no effects, and was used properly, this fact should be noted. It is very important to note any side effects of the drug, such as aggravating seizures, making the patient unsteady or drowsy, causing behavior problems or allergic reactions. It is also important to note true drug allergies so that these potentially dangerous reactions are not triggered again. Symptoms suggesting that the drug may have been too strong mean only that the drug may be retried at a lower dosage. Not only does a good drug history aid in selection of management approaches, it helps in the counseling of the parent and the patient regarding possible responses, reactions, and drugs to avoid.

Possible Causes (See Chapter 4)

A full review of the family may reveal seizures in relatives. If the relative's seizures are similar to the patients and if there is no apparent cause, the seizure disorder may be inherited. A full review of the pregnancy and birth period as well as past and present medical problems, head injuries, or possible exposures to drugs or poisonous substances may reveal insults leading to the development of an acquired seizure problem. Screening for previous episodes of fainting, unexplained falling, headaches, colic, staring, breath-holding, febrile seizures, or nightmares may reveal previous unrecognized seizure manifestations. Sometimes it is of value to request the actual birth records, for small clues in the chart may indicate insults to the brain during the crucial newborn period.

Developmental Disabilities

A review of the development as well as the present functioning of the patient is most important. The cause of the seizure may distort or delay the developmental milestones. The major areas to cover include motor and movement skills, speech and language, learning, and social-behavioral development. The parents' feelings about these functions also are important.

Motor and movement skills include strength, coordination, balance, tone, and handedness. Coordination includes both fine finger movements (as in buttoning, tying, cutting with scissors, coloring, and pencil work) and gross limb movements. Balance can cover unsteadiness in walking, sitting, or reaching. Unsteadiness can be related to the cause, the seizures, or the drugs used. The age of onset of a preference for the left or right hand is important. The story of the appearance of a definite preference for one hand over the other before one year of age, like the story of a left-handedness without a family history of other left-handers, suggests an increased risk for problems of the brain side opposite the nonpreferred hand.

Speech is the forming of words. It relates to the onset and normal development of saying clearly and correctly both the word sounds and the words. Language is the putting together of the words in order to transmit a thought. It describes the onset of the use of phrases and sentences, including appropriate word selection, order, grammar, and a smooth, fluent flow. Insults and seizure problems involving the left brain half, especially at an early age, result in an increased risk for problems in development of both speech and language. The difficulties may be caused by the seizures, even when they are nearly controlled. They may be due to the underlying cause or to the medication. Speech and language problems can become frustrating and thus become an additional handicap. Early remediation of such emerging problems may prevent this deterioration.

Learning problems and behavioral difficulties are both common consequences of seizures (see Chapters 12 and 13). Reviewing the patient's performance and behaviors at home, at school, or at work, including both achievement and problems, is most important. Progress and problems in social situations also should be considered. These items should not be looked at just during the initial examination; they should be reviewed at each succeeding re-evaluation, and progress or stagnation in development should be noted.

Deviations from expected development can become both frustrating and handicapping. Early recognition, leading to evaluation and follow-up remediation, may be able to prevent such problems from developing. The problem of epilepsy itself is enough of a handicap without the additional burdens of other difficulties. Monitoring ongoing performance and behavior is one of the best ways of determining the effectiveness of the management.

THE EXAMINATION

The main goals of the neurologic examination are to discover and investigate 1) any localized or abnormal findings, 2) any signs of increased pressure within the head, 3) any findings suggesting irritation to the brain or its coverings, 4) any clues that might suggest the possible cause of the seizures, and 5) any abnormal or delayed functions (alertness, speech, movement, behaviors, etc.) that might be due to the seizures, the cause of the seizures, or the medication.

The chances of finding abnormalities are somewhat related to the type of seizure disorder. The discovery of abnormalities in functioning in the examination and in the follow-up diagnostic studies is far more likely with focal seizures than with generalized seizures. With generalized seizures, the examination may be entirely normal unless there is a suspected cause. With multifocal seizures the likelihood of finding abnormalities is fairly high, but the causes of the abnormalities are often outside of the nervous system, and may include birthmarks, infections elsewhere in the body, enlargement of body organs, or problems in the lung, heart, or blood circulation. Sometimes these problems are inherited and sometimes they are acquired.

The time of the examination is most important. With seizures of acute onset there is great concern that the cause may be an acute, life-threatening insult. In a chronic disorder this is less likely, unless the problem is chronic and progressive. After any attack, acute or recurrent, the examination may show abnormal findings that are related to the aftereffects of the seizure, the medications used to stop the seizures, the cause of the seizures, or insults caused by the seizures. The effects of the seizure itself and of the medications used should gradually wear off over the succeeding hours or days, but they may remain up to several weeks. Symptoms and signs remaining three weeks after the last attack are significant and worrisome. Up to three weeks after the attack, symptoms that are becoming worse or the appearance of further symptoms also suggest that there is an active problem unless further seizures are occurring that have been overlooked.

The Acute Seizure

Immediately after a seizure, whether it be the first one or a severe attack in a patient known to have a seizure problem, the major purpose of the examination is to find and treat any problem that might either have caused the attack or that may be the result of the vigor of the convulsion. The immediate concerns are: 1) the vital signs (breathing, pulse, blood pressure, temperature), 2) the state of consciousness, 3) signs of trauma or increased pressure within the head, and 4) any indications of irritation to the coverings of the brain, the meninges.

Vital Signs The breathing rate, the pulse and heart rate, the blood pressure, and the temperature all may be increased after a vigorous seizure. The pulse rate and heartbeat also may be increased due to an infection, blood loss, breathing problems, anxiety, or medication. An irregular beat may be seen if there is some problem of the heart. The blood pressure may be low if the patient has lost blood or has received medication. The medical treatment for a long seizure may lead to low blood pressure. The patient may appear cold, clammy, pale, and shocky, with a fast heart rate in an effort to keep up. Conversely, the blood pressure can rise if the patient has a primary kidney problem or has increased pressure in the head. High blood pressure may be the cause or the result of the seizure, or another symptom of whatever caused the seizure.

Rapid and irregular breathing can be caused by an infection, blood loss, increased pressure in the head, brain damage, a chemical upset in the body or a poison, or an obstruction of the air passages. If the patient is blue, positioning the head and neck properly (see Chapter 8) and giving mouth-to-mouth resuscitation or oxygen may be helpful. An elevated temperature usually means an infection. The patient may feel hot to the touch and often tends to look pale or flushed.

State of Consciousness The patient may be fairly alert, but more often he appears confused and drowsy, or he can only be awakened with stimulation, or he is unarousable. The younger child tends to act dazed, irritable, and unresponsive, whereas the adolescent tends to act agitated, irritable, and unresponsive. The depressed consciousness may be the result of the seizure itself or the medication used to halt the seizure or the cause of the seizure.

Trauma and Pressure in the Head Trauma may be suspected from the findings of bruises, bumps, or cuts in the scalp, on the body surface, or in the mouth. Traumatic signs may be missed if the scalp is not carefully inspected. Head injuries may indicate potential problems within. In the younger child the brain can swell very rapidly to become life-threatening. Bleeding or brain swelling can both aggravate other problems and become dangerous problems themselves. The increasing pressure can lead to irregular breathing, a rise in the blood pressure, and a fall of the pulse rate, as well as a deeper degree of unconsciousness. A look at the back of the eyes through an ophthalmoscope may show patches of blood, engorgement of the blood vessels, and blurring of the end of the optic nerve where it enters into the eye. This finding is called papilledema, which means increased pressure in the head, although it doesn't tell why. Eye changes may be present at the exam or may develop within hours, although often the papilledema takes longer to show up. A difference in the size of the pupils, the failure of the pupils to become smaller when a light is shone into them, or the deviation of one or both eyes outward or inward are worrisome signs also. Other signs of significant head trauma are bruised swelling around both eyes, swelling of the eardrum or behind the ear, or the gushing of clear, sugar-containing watery fluid from the nose. These are signs suggestive of a skull fracture.

Signs of Meningeal Irritation

A stiff neck, especially if accompanied by a fever, suggests an infection of the brain coverings, the meninges. The tendency toward a guarding stiffness of the neck in meningitis is an early finding in the older child or adult, but it is a late finding in the younger child or infant. A stiff, guarding neck posture may also be seen if the neck has been strained or injured, or if the lymph nodes in the neck are sore and inflamed from an infection, or if there is pressure or a mass in the posterior and lower part of the head.

A red or ruptured and pus-leaking eardrum may be found. An ear infection may trigger a seizure or it may lead to meningitis or a brain abscess that results in seizures. Fluid behind the ear also indicates infection, unless the fluid is bloody purple-red, as with trauma. Not only are ear disturbances frequently seen with young seizure patients, but they can lead to hearing problems and further handicaps if they are not discovered and treated.

These are the immediate concerns in evaluating the acute seizure for the existence of a life-threatening cause that may require immediate action if found. Even the patient with a known seizure disorder may have any of these problems. The seizure does not protect him against meningitis or head trauma, and, indeed, it may make him more prone to experience the latter. It is always a good idea to check the patient for any signs of a new head trauma whenever the patient is evaluated.

The Main Examination

The aims of the examination are to determine the cause of the seizure and to detect any additional problems. Subtle problems such as cysts, vascular malformations, or tumors may not be apparent on the initial examination; signs may begin to emerge on later examination. The three main areas of the examination include: 1) the general appearance, 2) the physical examination, and 3) the neurologic examination.

General Appearance Overgrowth of a body part may be due to a vascular problem or to a neurocutaneous (nerve and skin) disorder called neurofibromatosis. Underdevelopment may be due to a congenital problem, damage to the peripheral nerves, or brain damage. Abnormal sizes of half the body can sometimes be seen with tumors of the kidneys or adrenal glands. One type of size difference is parietal or sensory hemiplegia, in which one limb is smaller than the other. The size differences can be noted when the large digits (e.g., thumbs, toes) are compared. The patient tends to hold the limb in odd postures and seems unaware of how to use it. The limb is neither as stiff or as weak as it appears, and indeed the reflexes may be fairly normal. A good sensory examination reveals that the person may have a sensory loss. The insult usually occurs in early infancy or even before birth.

Abnormal posturing can give clues to brain damage. In the usual hemiplegia (half-body weakness), the arm is held close to the body in a bent position with the leg tending to be stretched out and stiff in usage. This suggests damage to the motor areas of the opposite brain half. If both sides of the body are like this, the so-called "decorticate posture" suggests widespread damage, involving especially the cortical brain covering and underlying areas. If the arms are stretched out and stiff like the legs, the problem involves the entire brain halves of both sides in the more severe "decerebrate posture." Twisting and jerky, unsteady, or distorted posturing suggest disturbances deep in the brain or brainstem.

A head that is too large suggests that 1) the skull may be abnormally thick, 2) there may be a collection of blood or tumor masses within, 3) the brain may be too large (possibly due to the accumulation of abnormal substances), or 4) the normal flow of cerebrospinal fluid may be blocked, resulting in hydrocephalus. The skin may be stretched tight and the scalp vessels may be overly filled with blood. The eyes may deviate abnormally. In infants, the soft spot (the fontanelle) may seem overly filled with fluid, to the point of being tense and bulging. The suture spaces between the skull bone may be wider than normal.

A small or peculiarly shaped head suggests damage or underdevelopment of part or all of the brain beneath. A bulging area may overlie a sac of fluid or a mass. Infants with large heads or abnormally shaped heads can be examined in a dark room by holding a very bright flashlight to the head. A diffuse excessive glow suggests hydrocephalus, whereas a localized glow suggests a cyst or a sac of fluid. Another cause of abnormal head shape is early closure of the suture between two adjacent skull bones. The suture may close because the brain is not growing enough to keep it open, or it may close abnormally early, leaving the brain with no place to grow unless other areas of the head can overgrow. The head may end up being long and narrow, short and flat, or asymmetrical.

The development of both the face and the brain are under similar influences. Abnormal facial appearances may be related to abnormal brain formation. Eyes spaced too widely apart may be seen when the front bones of the skull do not unite correctly, or in some cases of hydrocephalus. Eyes that are too close together, sometimes with the eyebrows joined as one, when accompanied by a split in the middle of the lip (rather than a cleft lip to the side, as is usually seen), may be associated with a malformed brain. Some types of genetic problems, such as mongolism, may present with a fairly typical and recognizable face. Seizures are more apt to be a complication of malformation problems than genetic disorders unless the latter condition and its consequent insult to the brain produce a seizure disorder.

The midline of the body extends from the lower end of the backbone up the spine and over the middle of the head to end at the base of the nose.

This is the area where the nervous system, which originates from the same tissue as the skin, developed and sank beneath the surface, to be covered over by the skin and underlying bone. Sometimes this closure is incomplete, leaving anything from a small hole to a gaping chasm. A closure defect can occur at either end of the midline. The defect may be marked by a lump of misplaced tissue, a brown or red birthmark, a tuft of abnormal hair, a defect in the underlying bone, or, if larger, a sac of the nervous system bulging outward. If the problem is at the head end, malformations and seizures are apt to occur; if it is at the tail end, as with a meningomyelocele, there may also be hydrocephalus and possibly seizures due to the complications of care.

Since the nervous system and the skin originated from a common source, birth defects, such as red vascular markings, brown café au lait patches, and white achromic patches, as well as lumps of abnormally developed tissue, may involve both the skin and the nervous system. These are called neurocutaneous (nerve-skin) disorders. The true spot-and-lump disease, called neurofibromatosis, may present with brown spots of the skin and lumps in the skin and on the nervous system. A more severe problem is that of both brown and white spots of the skin and lumps in the brain and other body organs. This is called tuberous sclerosis. Other neurocutaneous problems include those of vascular red marks of the skin and of the nervous system. Sturge-Weber syndrome is one such example, with a large red birthmark involving the middle or upper part of half the face and half the brain, with x-rays revealing related calcifications on the brain surface. These are the most common neurocutaneous syndromes associated with seizures.

Skin lesions may give clues to other body problems. Petechiae are small purple-red hemorrhages that suggest a bleeding problem, as does spontaneous bruising not caused by trauma. Bright hemorrhages located beneath the fingernails can come from particles of infection carried in the bloodstream. Rashes may relate to an infection or an allergic reaction. Liver or kidney problems may show up as swelling of the face or puffiness of the limbs.

General Examination In the general examination, special attention is paid to three areas, 1) the heart, the lungs, and the blood circulation, 2) possible sources of infection, and 3) any enlarged body organs.

A large or extra-active heart, an irregular heartbeat, or abnormal heart sounds, called murmurs, heard in listening to the heart, suggest a malformation or an infection. Abnormal sounds (called bruits) heard over a blood vessel elsewhere in the body suggest a narrowing, an obstruction, or a malformation. It is most important to listen for these sounds in the head of a seizure patient because the cause of the seizures might be a vascular malformation of the brain. With heart diseases or with inflammations of the blood vessels, small chunks of blood clot may form and break off into the bloodstream, blocking off blood vessels of the brain and causing a stroke. In patients with chronic lung problems or with malformed hearts, the blood may become very thick in order to carry enough oxygen. Sometimes this thick blood blocks a blood vessel of the brain, causing a stroke. Dehydration can also cause this.

If the lungs are not absorbing oxygen well, if the heart is deformed, or if the heartbeat is irregular, there may not be an adequate delivery of oxygen-carrying blood to the brain. The patient may experience episodes of blueness; he may tire very easily. Severe but brief episodes of lack of a good blood flow to the brain, as with fainting, low blood pressure, or irregular heartbeat, can lead to an acute lack of oxygen in the brain. The patient not only loses consciousness, he may also experience a few convulsive movements as the brain cells protest against the oxygen starvation.

An infection somewhere in the body, such as in the ear, nose, throat, chest, lymph glands of the neck, or joints, can cause a seizure in a young child due to the resulting high temperature from the infection. The infection may spread to the brain and brain coverings, resulting in seizures due to meningitis or a brain abscess.

Enlargement of the liver, the spleen, or the lymph glands may be seen with some infections. Enlargement of the liver and spleen can also be seen in heart failure. More often this is seen when there is a congenital disorder of the handling of certain body substances, resulting in accumulation of irritating chemicals in these enlarged organs and also in the brain. Sometimes abnormal body metabolism of these chemicals will show up as abnormal odors; some drugs and poisons may also produce peculiar body or breath smells.

The Neurologic Examination The goals of a good neurologic examination are to note: 1) any asymmetrical or localizing disturbances of function, 2) any abnormal functions, 3) any signs of increased pressure, or 4) any indications of irritation to the brain or its coverings. Mental, emotional, and language functions are also evaluated. The neurologic exam is often divided into four major areas, consisting of motor-movements, sensation, including vision and the other special senses, language, and an estimate of the alertness, intelligence, and emotional status.

The motor system exam notes the fullness, smoothness, coordination, and strength of both fine and large movements of the limbs and digits, the face, the tongue and throat, and the eyes. Abnormal movements, twitches, tremors, and unsteadiness are all looked for. Various reflexes are checked by stimulating the skin or deeper structures and noting the speed and degree of response. For example, striking a muscle tendon with a rubber hammer produces a responsive movement of the limb. The Babinski sign is an important abnormal finding: if upon stroking the outer edge of the sole of the foot the examiner notes an initial raising of the big toe and spreading outward of the other toes, he should suspect some significant disturbance of the motor system of the brain. Slowed, awkward, uncontrolled, or unsteady movements or tone abnormalities, such as floppiness or stiffness in movements, are noted and localized.

The sensory examination is divided into three types of sensations: 1) simple or crude sensations, such as pain, touch, temperature, etc.; 2) complex or discrimination sensations requiring recognition of the stimulus or choosing between alternatives such as big-small, warm-cold, up-down, coarse-smooth, etc.; and 3) special sensations, such as hearing, vision, taste, and smell. Crude sensations are handled deep within the brain. Sensations requiring recognition of forms, shapes, or traced figures or requiring a choice between two similar stimuli are the sensations registered on the brain cortical surface over the posterior half, the parietal lobe of the brain.

Of the special sensations, vision receives the most emphasis. The visual fields are tested, one eye at a time, by seeing how far to the edges of vision the patient can see a small object being wiggled while he looks straight ahead. A section or wedge of blindness may be seen if a defect of the brain is present; the defective vision may appear in both eye fields. Sometimes this condition can be discovered by testing both sides simultaneously; the patient may ignore one finger and recognize the other when both fingers are wiggled simultaneously, whereas when they are moved separately he can recognize either. Another approach is to pull a piece of striped cloth from left to right and then from right to left in front of the patient's eyes. The eyes should drift along with the cloth and then jerk back to looking ahead normally, over and over. These vision tests evaluate not only the receptive cortical area of the surface of the occipital lobe in the very back of the brain, but also the deeper visual pathways that run beneath the parietal and temporal lobes.

Motor and sensory findings are compared from side to side and against normal expectations. An asymmetry suggests a problem with the brain half opposite the abnormal finding, with motor problems in the mid-portions of the brain and sensory abnormalities in the back half.

Language and intelligence are closely related. Language functions usually come from the left brain half, whereas intelligence is more widespread. Observing how well the patient understands what he hears and reads and how well he speaks or writes both spontaneously and when presented with specific tasks to perform is used to check this. Speech, the forming of words, may be interfered with by any movement problem. Such items as drawing, dressing, telling time, knowing directions, and building simple designs tend to be functions arising from the other side of the brain than that used for language. These functions can be tested by asking questions and by getting the patient to draw. Memory can be tested by asking the patient to count, to recite the alphabet, to recall addresses, phone numbers, simple facts, and recent events, or to repeat back a series of numbers or a short sentence.

Alertness and emotional behavior are evaluated more by observing the patient during the overall examination than by direct testing. Depending on his age and intelligence, the patient should know who he is, where he is, and the approximate time, date, or season. His attentiveness, cooperation, and overall interaction with the examiner lead to the final impression.

Specific Focal Disorders

If the seizure disorder has been localized to a specific portion of the brain, at each examination the evaluation should be more intense for functions related to that part of the brain. The left brain half usually relates to language processes; if the seizure originates from this half, close attention must be paid to speech and understanding. The frontal portion of the brain is rather difficult to evaluate since its functions tend to be rather vague, including such skills as planning, social behavior, and some emotional aspects. The back half of the frontal lobe is the motor strip; seizures from here mean that close attention must be paid to muscle strength and tone, reflexes, and coordination. Behind this, on the surface of the parietal lobe, is where sensory recognition and choosing between similar stimuli are located; these functions must be evaluated if the patient has sensory seizures. Just testing the sensations of pain, temperature, and touch is not enough; these sensations are not registered on the surface where the seizures originate. Vision is processed in the very back of the brain, the occipital lobe, although the pathways travel beneath the parietal lobe and loop around into the temporal lobe on their way back. Nicks and chunks out of the visual field may help to indicate problems in the occipital lobe, the deep parietal lobe, or the deep temporal lobe. Other ways of checking out temporal lobe function include testing memory, understanding, and to some extent learning skills. Immediately above the temporal lobe is a major collection of blood vessels; it is a good idea to listen carefully for any bruits in this area, especially if the seizure is a temporal lobe problem.

Seeing a Seizure

It is very valuable to observe a seizure. Some seizures can and should be stimulated as part of the examination. For example, if a sudden sound or a flashing light seems to trigger the seizure, the examiner should attempt to mimic this stimulus, hoping that a short seizure will result. The attack may be a stare, a pause, a jerk, or a few jerks, but it is seldom more unless the stimulus is continued.

Hyperventilation may bring out absence attacks. Having the patient breathe deeply for about three minutes requires much encouragement and the promise of water as soon as the test is completed. If a spell appears, the patient should be told a word to remember and repeat back after the attack. A younger child may be more willing to try this if he is repeatedly asked to blow hard enough to bend a piece of paper. Hyperventilation may also produce other unpleasant symptoms and the patient should be asked about these. His reactions may give clues to other causes of the attacks.

CONCLUSION

The initial examination searches for causes and related problems associated with the seizure. At each follow-up re-examination these areas must be screened, with special emphasis on functions related to the seizure focus or in follow-up of previously noted abnormalities. The patient should also be checked for any possible problems arising from bad attacks in the interval. The examinations should also note any signs of drug reactions (see Chapter 10) such as drowsiness, drunkenness, or other reactions. All these observations, when thoughtfully considered, can be used to determine and correctly interpret laboratory tests in order to confirm or correct clinical concerns and to select proper management of the seizure problem and any other problems identified.

REFERENCES AND FURTHER READING

Castle, C. F., and L. S. Fishman. 1973. Seizures. Pediatr. Clin. North Am. 20: 819-835.

Commission for Control of Epilepsy and Its Consequences. 1977. Plan for Nationwide Action on Epilepsy, 4 Volumes. Office of Scientific and Health Reports. National Institute of Neurological and Communicative Disorders and Stroke, Bldg. 3, Room 8A406, Bethesda, Maryland. 248 pp. (Vol. I.)

DeMyer, W. 1969. Technique of the Neurologic Examination. McGraw-Hill Book Company, New York. 442 pp.

Lennox, W. G. 1960. Epilepsy and Related Disorders. Little, Brown & Company, Boston. 1168 pp.

Mayo Clinic, Department of Neurology. 1976. Clinical Examinations in Neurology, 4th Ed. W. B. Saunders Company, Philadelphia. 285 pp.

Penfield, W., and H. Jasper. 1954. Epilepsy and the Functional Anatomy of the Human Brain. Little, Brown & Company, Boston. 896 pp.

Solomon, G. E., and F. Plum. 1976. Clinical Management of Seizures. W. B. Saunders Company, Philadelphia. 152 pp.

6
MIMICS OF SEIZURE DISORDERS

Any recurring abnormal movement, sensation, behavior, stare, or other brain function that begins abruptly, lasts but a brief time, and resolves rapidly back to normal might be a seizure. It may also be some other type of brain disturbance, such as a temporary decrease in the flow of blood to the brain, or an emotional reaction, or some other problem that produces symptoms similar to those of a seizure. The brainwave test (EEG) may be abnormal, but the abnormality may not relate to the symptoms. A beneficial response to an anticonvulsant drug does not prove that the spell was a seizure, for these medications do have other beneficial effects; they are used for other problems of other systems in addition to those of the brain. Some of the other useful effects include the controlling of excessive activity, the stimulation of sluggish activity, the calming of overly sensitive reactions, the stabilizing of unstable systems, and the relaxing of spasms in various body parts. Some of these drugs may even give partial relief from pain, help control fever, or promote healing. For example, phenobarbital also can be used for sedation, for tranquilization, for itching, for fever, or in asthma, ulcers, colitis, yellow jaundice, and in many other ways for disorders that are clearly not seizures.

Key points in differentiating between a seizure and some other type of spell are based on the appearance, the time, and the duration of the attack; on the state of consciousness during and immediately after the spell; on the relationship of the attack to surrounding stimuli; and the patient's own emotional feelings about the attack. A true seizure usually begins fairly abruptly, with brief, if any, warning (the aura usually lasts less than a minute); the seizure has fairly characteristic symptoms and signs; and it resolves fairly rapidly, although the aftereffects may linger. The main attack is brief, usually lasting only seconds to minutes. Consciousness is disturbed during and frequently after the attack. The patient often is somewhat forgetful of the spell afterward. True seizures usually are not significantly influenced by events or stimuli during the attack. Often the seizure patient is ashamed of these attacks. There are exceptions to these tendencies.

A spell that may look like a seizure often is rather vague in both onset and resolution. The symptoms during the attack may or may not resemble any of the known seizure manifestations or they may be bizarre and unlike any usual seizure picture. The patient usually remains conscious and alert both during and after the spell and tends to remember the spell much better than he will admit. These spells are often significantly longer in duration than a seizure, lasting minutes to hours. The patient is more apt to feel indifferent, annoyed, anxious, or fascinated by the attacks rather than to be ashamed of them. Obviously there are specific exceptions to these trends also. (A listing of spells that may mimic certain seizures is given in Table 6.1.)

For convenience, the cluster of symptomatic attacks that may or may not be seizures can be divided into five groups: 1) those attacks characterized by strange thoughts, peculiar behaviors, or emotional disturbances; 2) those attacks characterized by disturbances of a sensation or special sense, often accompanied by headache; 3) the staring episodes; 4) episodes of loss of consciousness, sometimes followed by brief convulsive jerking or stiffening; and 5) those episodes characterized by abnormal movements or posturing, such as sudden jerks in infants, attacks of recurrent, fairly localized movements, or whole body attacks of abnormal movements or posturing.

PECULIAR BEHAVIORS, DISTURBED EMOTIONS, OR STRANGE THOUGHTS

There are numerous problems, in addition to complex focal seizures, that can cause episodes of disturbed thoughts, emotions, or behaviors. These include the emotional disorders and behavioral difficulties, disturbances in the body chemistry, such as low blood sugar, interruptions in the blood flow to the brain, triggered discharges from an overly sensitive autonomic nervous system, allergic reactions, or the effects of drugs and poisons.

Feelings of anxiety or terror may result from any of these factors. If the cause is a seizure, the onset is abrupt and unrelated to anything happening at the time. The attack is brief, lasting usually only seconds to minutes. The patient is confused during, and often for a time after, the attack. He may wander aimlessly or at times run. He does not remember the details of the attack clearly although he may recall some fragments. Non-convulsive spells tend to build up less abruptly; these spells last longer. Usually the patient remains fairly alert during and after a spell, with good recall if he is willing to try.

Nightmares and night terrors may be seizure symptoms but more often are related to anxiety or emotional turmoil. A child who has had a bad

Table 6.1. Spells that look like seizures

Seizure	Condition That May Mimic Seizures
Generalized Seizures	
Generalized Motor	Hysteria, Breath-holding, Faints
Myoclonic Jerks	Tics, Chorea, Falls, "Bad Eyes"
Infantile Spasms	Startle, Colic, Temper tantrums
Akinetic Drops	Falls, Faints
Absence Stares	Daydreaming, Drugs
Focal Seizures	
Simple	
Motor	Tics, Chorea
Sensory	Migraine, Blood flow problems, Ear problems
Autonomic	Migraine, Ear problems, Flu, Anxiety
Complex	
Psychomotor	Emotions, Behaviors, Hyperventilation
Affect	Drug usage
Cognitive	
Consciousness	Faint, Breath-holding, Unseen trauma

dream tends to sit up rather suddenly in wide-eyed terror after he has been in a deep sleep. He may scream in fright. His heart rate and breathing are fast. He cannot be awakened. After a few minutes he falls back to a calmer sleep. He does not remember the event. By comparison, seizures tend to occur in the light stages of sleep. The pulse and breathing are not as fast. The seizure patient may be able to remember part of the attack. He too is hard to awaken.

Anxiety can lead to attacks of over-breathing. The patient often is not aware of his hyperventilation. He may complain of dizziness and of tingling sensations around his mouth and in his fingers and toes. He may seem out of contact, but he is fully alert and can remember the attack. These episodes last longer than a typical seizure. They tend to resolve slowly; breathing into a paper bag may hasten the resolution. Sometimes the hyperventilation can trigger an absence seizure.

Anger outbursts, including temper tantrums, rage reactions, and aggressive acting out, have often been confused with temporal lobe seizures. There is an increased incidence of these episodes in patients known to have temporal lobe seizures, but these behavioral attacks are not true seizures. Unlike a seizure, the behavioral outburst is usually triggered by something or someone, although to others the irritation may seem minor. The outburst may sometimes be planned. It usually is directed at the source of irritation. The pattern of the episode may vary from time to time. The patient remains totally alert during and after the spell, which usually lasts longer than a seizure. He remembers the events of the attack although he may deny this as he contritely claims innocence. These attacks may build up slowly or appear suddenly. In a true seizure, the confused patient does not attack any specific thing or person, although he may accidently harm anything that gets in his way during the seizure.

Hysterical episodes of bizarre behaviors can be mistaken for seizures. An immature mind may mimic the actions of somebody else in order to gain attention. Often there is a significant degree of some form of movement in the attack. Hysterical seizures are discussed later on in this chapter.

Some patients experience sudden, brief outbursts of laughter or occasionally tears without any apparent reason. These outbursts may be a rare form of complex focal seizures called gelastic seizures. Such an attack is unpredictable, unstimulated by anything around the patient, and unaccompanied by an appropriate facial expression of joy or sorrow. These attacks are typically abrupt in onset, short in duration, and resolve quickly. The patient appears dazed or confused both during and after the attack. He may pause in his activities. His memory of the attack is often poor. Most outbursts of sudden emotional behavior are just that, and no more. Another rare problem that begins as a pure emotional outburst is cataplexy. The emotional outburst may cause the patient to become so weak that he falls to the ground, as if paralyzed. This is often related to an abnormal tendency to fall asleep called narcolepsy. Neither of these conditions is a seizure.

The autonomic nervous system controls the autonomic functions of our body, such as heartbeat, blood circulation, breathing, blood pressure, gastrointestinal function, and kidney function, to name but a few. Sometimes this system is overly sensitive and swings erratically from too much of one type of discharge to too much of another. Such disorders as migraine headaches, dizziness, high blood pressure, irregular heartbeat, some forms of asthma, colic, low blood sugars, periodic vomiting, stomach cramps, or diarrhea are but a few symptoms of this disfunction. Other problems include rare tumors that irritate the autonomic nervous system, as well as some drugs, some poisons, and many types of emotional reactions, including anxiety. The patient may appear flushed or pale. He is usually alert, anxious, and perhaps irritable. He may be jumpy and jittery, nauseated, and sweaty or tremulous. These attacks mimic autonomic seizures but they tend to begin slowly, last longer, and resolve gradually. The patient remembers these attacks quite well.

SENSORY SYMPTOMS, SOMETIMES WITH HEADACHES

Some patients complain of feelings of warmth, coldness, tingling, heaviness, or disturbed touch in some part of their bodies. Most often this is due to pressure on or stretching of a nerve. The patient becomes aware of this, changes his position, and the sensation gradually fades. Similar symptoms can be seen with hyperventilation, although the location of the tingling is more vague. Sensory disturbances can originate from the posterior half of the brain. The causes include not only sensory seizures but also interference with blood flow, as happens with a migraine headache or stroke, or some other irritation to this area. Seizures tend to last seconds to minutes, whereas other problems usually last longer.

A patient with migraine headaches may first note a personality change, dizziness, nausea, jitteriness, peculiar sensations, or sparkling lights dancing before his eyes. He may become sensitive to sound and light. His speech, his coordination, or his vision may be distorted. He may appear pale or flushed. After 5 to 15 minutes he may begin to develop a pounding headache, often located on one side of the head, as the other symptoms begin to lessen. Vomiting may bring relief. A seizure may also be followed by a headache, but the entire attack is much quicker than a migraine. After a seizure, a stroke, or a migraine, the patient tends to feel fatigued and often confused.

Strokes, like migraine headaches, can happen at any age. The attack comes abruptly, with a loss of function or a strange sensation that may improve after a few seconds or may continue to resolve for a matter of hours to days. Sometimes the insult of a stroke may trigger a brief convulsive reaction. The patient is usually quite aware and able to recall the episode, although he may seem confused.

Some children experience episodes of dizziness, nausea, and vomiting that may last minutes to days and that tend to recur. The child remains alert, although he looks and is uncomfortable during the attack. An excessive discharge of the autonomic nervous system may be noted. Children tend to outgrow these benign paroxysmal vertigo spells although they may later develop migraine symptoms. Adults can experience similar bouts of dizziness in which they tend to fall to one side. There is usually a problem of the inner ear. The patient tends to be deaf on that side. Temporal lobe seizures may resemble these spells but are much briefer in duration.

A child may experience recurring bouts of vomiting or abdominal pain. These conditions have sometimes been called abdominal epilepsy or abdominal migraines because they tend to respond to some of the sedative effects of anticonvulsant drugs. Unlike seizures, these attacks last much longer. They are not accompanied by any disturbance of consciousness. Recurring cramping pains or sharp excruciating distress is probably never a seizure. The abdominal discomfort of seizures is usually not painful.

STARING EPISODES

A child may stare because he is daydreaming, uninterested, overwhelmed by a task, trying to think of an answer, under the influence of drugs, or having an absence seizure. Absence attacks usually last less than a minute. The patient is totally out of contact. The attacks begin abruptly and often end abruptly, although occasionally there may be some after-confusion. The attack is often not remembered. During the attacks the pupils may enlarge and the eyelids may flutter. The attacks may occur frequently during the day. With non-seizure stares, the attacks are longer and more vague in onset. The patient is preoccupied but not unconscious. He can be aroused from the attack, although he may have to reorient himself to what he was supposed to be doing.

LOSS OF CONSCIOUSNESS

Loss of consciousness, often with falling, can be caused by a seizure, an abrupt lessening of the blood flow to the brain (as with a faint), an irregular heartbeat, blockage of a blood vessel, or breath-holding spells. Other causes may include a fall, unobserved head truma, or the previously mentioned weakness, which may be associated with laughter. With non-seizure problems the patient experiences some dizziness or light-headedness. His vision fades and he slumps to the floor, but he tries to protect himself during the fall. With a seizure there may be only a brief warning before the patient abruptly falls, without trying to protect himself.

In infants and young children, breath-holding spells may mimic seizures. These are reflex reactions to pain, fright, or anger. The initial crying ceases and the child stops breathing. The heart may slow down or it may speed up. The patient either turns blue or pale white. He then faints. If the attack is severe, as with fainting episodes in an older person, some stiffening, jerking, or wetting of his clothes may occur; he may be drowsy and fatigued upon recovery. With seizures, the loss of consciousness and stiffening or jerking come before the interference with breathing and the color changes.

If a fainting episode is prolonged or if the patient hits his head as he falls, the insult to the brain may produce some secondary convulsive movements, especially if there is a tendency toward seizures. Fainting spells usually occur when the patient is upright, whereas seizures can occur in any position.

ABNORMAL MOVEMENTS: JERKS, STIFFENING, OR FALLING

Abnormal movements can be confused with seizure disorders. Three types of abnormal movements may be considered: 1) jerks or tremors in infants, 2) repeated movements, often localized to a part of the body, and 3) major movement disturbances, usually involving the entire body.

Jerks and Tremors in Infants

Jerking movements in infants may be due to colic or stomach cramps, temper, a startle response to a loud stimulus, or myoclonic spasms. Rarely, head bobbing may be due to eye problems. In the ominous but brief myoclonic spasms of infancy, the child tends to be only momentarily unconscious, whereas with the other problems, which last longer, the patient is usually preoccupied with pain, anger, or fright. Colic, cramps, and myoclonic spasms may occur in clusters, but those symptoms related to the intestinal tract are fairly rhythmic and slower in nature. Because of the poor outlook and possibility of beneficial treatment for myoclonic spasms in infancy, if there is any question that the attacks may be seizures, the child should be checked with a brainwave test (EEG).

Repeated and Usually Local Movements

The most common mimics of focal motor seizures are the emotional nervous twitches and tics. With these spells the patient remains alert and unconcerned. The attack may consist of eye blinking, facial grimacing or twitching, shoulder shrugging, or various throat sounds. These manifestations do not interfere with his activities; he can put them off if he wishes. The spells usually relate to external stresses. These features help to differentiate a nervous habit from a seizure.

Some young patients may present with episodes of tilting or holding of the head to one side. The episodes may last minutes to days. The patient may tend to fall to the side. He may be nauseated, pale, and sweaty. Occasionally the eyes may show jerky movements. This condition is called benign paroxysmal torticollis (twisted neck), which like benign paroxysmal vertigo (dizziness) may be an early form of migraine headaches.

Eye disorders can cause peculiar head movements that can be mistaken for seizures. An imbalance of the eye muscles can cause the child to tilt his head when he is looking at something. Poor vision can lead to bobbing and shaking movements of the head during infancy. This is called spasmus nutans. Often the eyes are out of balance. Not infrequently, to-and-fro nystagmoid jerky movements may be seen. A rare problem is oculomotor apraxia. The child cannot voluntarily move his eyes back and forth although the eye muscles and nerves are normal. The child is able to move his eyes back and forth by stimulating certain reflexes. He does this by blinking his eyes and jerking his head to the side. This may look like a seizure but it isn't.

Major Movement Disturbances, Usually Generalized

The most common mimics of generalized seizures include hysterical emotional attacks, fainting (with brief convulsive movements), and occasionally some episodic movement disorders.

Hysterical emotional attacks are vague, variable, and often bizarre. They may not resemble any typical seizure pattern. The onset is often not as abrupt as in a seizure attack. The patient remains fully alert. He can recall what was said and done during the attack if he can be tricked into admitting this. The attacks seem closely related to events and people around him. These spells may be lengthy, sometimes waxing and waning in character. The patient may arch backward to an extreme, with strange thrashing movements of his limbs, or he may display some other type of bizarre movement. The eyes may be held tightly closed and the eyelids may quiver. The patient rarely hurts himself during an attack and almost never wets himself. He may react to painful or unpleasant stimuli by avoidance efforts. The attack may end abruptly, with either abrupt or gradual recovery. When the attack has ended, the patient appears surprisingly alert and unbothered by the episode despite the wildness of the spell. He seems more unconcerned than ashamed of the attack.

Hysterical seizures can occur in people with or without known seizures. The attack is a subconscious means of either getting extra attention or avoiding something unpleasant. Thus the "seizure" is of benefit to the patient. In diagnosing an hysterical or conversion reaction, as it is sometimes called, it is important to determine where the patient learned to mimic a seizure, and how it benefits him.

Movement disorders are rarely mistaken for seizures. These problems include the irregular jerks and flings of chorea, the slow twisting movements of athetosis, or the distorted, twisted, frozen postures of dystonia. Sometimes brief attacks of choreoathetosis or torsion spasms of dystonia may be triggered by certain stresses. These attacks may run in a family. The degree of a sudden disability is so striking that it may be thought to be a seizure, but the patient remains fully conscious. The attack may last seconds to hours or longer. There may be some degree of an ongoing movement disorder in addition to these major spasms.

CONCLUSION

No matter what the symptoms, the rate of onset and recovery, the duration of the spell, the state of consciousness during the spell, the degree of recall after the spell, and the relationship of the spell to the surroundings may help to differentiate non-epileptic spells and true seizures. Seizures usually are of abrupt onset, shorter duration, and a greater disturbance of consciousness than other types of attacks. Often the course of the attack may go on to more familiar symptoms related to a seizure or to some other problems. This helps with the diagnosis. More typical seizure manifestations may appear. The question then may arise whether this is entirely a convulsive disorder or whether the seizure is a secondary response to some other type of spell. The final decision may depend on the findings of the brain-wave test (EEG) and other studies.

REFERENCES AND FURTHER READINGS

Dreifuss, F. E. 1975. The differential diagnosis of partial seizures with complex symptomatology. In: J. K. Penry and D. D. Daly (eds.), Advances in Neurology, Vol. 11, Chapter 9. Raven Press, New York. 13 pp.

Gomez, M. R., and D. W. Klass. 1972. Seizures and other paroxysmal disorders in infants and children. Current Problems in Pediatrics, Vol. 2, Nos. 6 and 7. Year Book Medical Publishers Inc., Chicago. 38 pages each.

Livingston, S. 1972. Comprehensive Management of Epilepsy in Infancy, Childhood and Adolescence. Charles C Thomas, Springfield, Illinois. 657 pp.

Singer, H. S., and J. M. Freeman. 1975. Seizures in adolescents. Med. Clin. North Am. 59:1461-1472.

Solomon, G. E., and F. Plum. 1976. Clinical Management of Seizures. W. B. Saunders Company, Philadelphia. 152 pp.

7
LABORATORY DIAGNOSIS

With suspected seizure disorders the diagnostic aims are: 1) to confirm, question, or correct the clinical impressions; 2) to discover a cause whenever possible; and 3) to identify any other problems. Minimal standards of medical care have been identified but there is no single approach that can be used with all patients. A good evaluation suggests what tests are needed, what the results mean, and what management might be most helpful.

An intensive study may be indicated when the seizures have just begun, are changing in character, are becoming worse despite good management, or appear in a newborn or very young infant. Chronic, unchanging seizure problems usually do not require vigorous diagnostic study.

The type of seizure suggests possible causes and consequently the most appropriate studies. Focal seizures are often caused by focal brain irritations, active or old. The studies are more apt to include those tests that identify focal structural changes in parts of the brain. Generalized or multifocal seizures are more apt to be caused by problems affecting the entire brain, such as infections, chemical problems, or poisons. Thorough blood and perhaps spinal fluid studies should be pursued, especially in the acute period of the attack. An outline of laboratory studies employed in diagnosis is given in Figure 7.1.

HOSPITALIZATION

The patient is hospitalized for observation of peculiar seizure problems, for special studies, for the beginning of complicated management approaches, for support after a severe or prolonged attack or its complications, or for the care of any severe reactions to therapy. Otherwise both the evaluation and the therapy are accomplished on an out-patient basis.

A simple work-up takes 3 to 7 days or less. Initiating seizure control usually takes days to weeks. A full rehabilitative program may take weeks to months. For complicated cases, a referral to a center specializing in epilepsy may be best. Hospitalization may be prolonged by complications in diagno-

68   Learning About Epilepsy

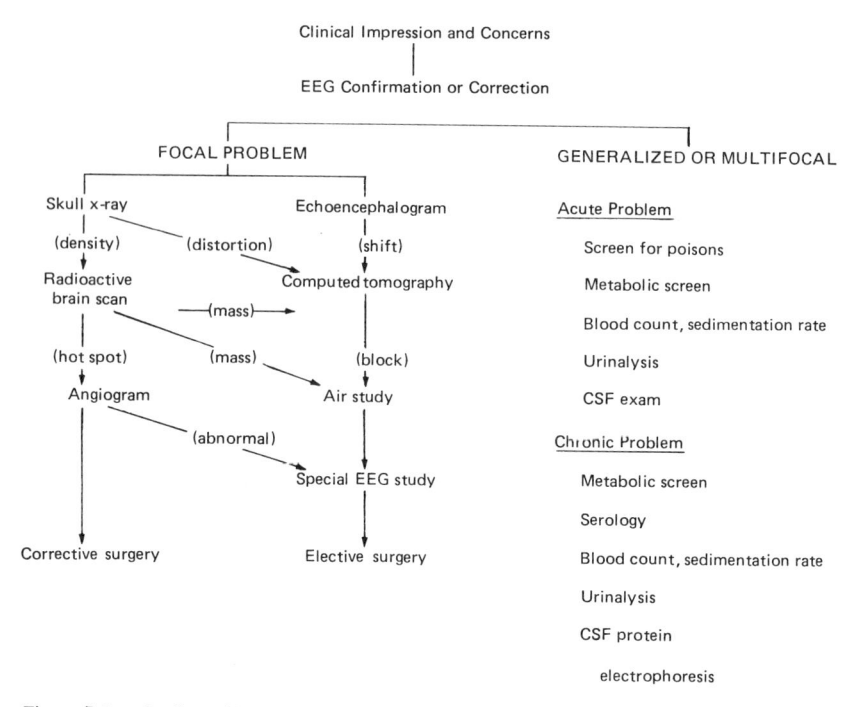

```
                    Clinical Impression and Concerns
                                 |
                    EEG Confirmation or Correction
        ┌────────────────────────┴────────────────────────┐
              FOCAL PROBLEM                    GENERALIZED OR MULTIFOCAL
        ┌────────────┴────────────┐
   Skull x-ray              Echoencephalogram         Acute Problem
       |                                              Screen for poisons
   (density)    (distortion)      (shift)
       ↓             ↓              ↓                 Metabolic screen
   Radioactive              Computed tomography
   brain scan   ──(mass)──→                           Blood count, sedimentation rate
       |                                              Urinalysis
   (hot spot)     (mass)          (block)
       ↓             ↘              ↓                 CSF exam
   Angiogram                    Air study
                                                      Chronic Problem
                  (abnormal)       ↓
                              Special EEG study       Metabolic screen
                                   |
                                   ↓                  Serology
   Corrective surgery        Elective surgery         Blood count, sedimentation rate
                                                      Urinalysis
                                                      CSF protein
                                                        electrophoresis
```

Figure 7.1. Outline of laboratory studies performed in diagnosis of epilepsy.

sis or management and by the need for additional studies or for further care of problems identified in the evaluation. When all the studies are completed, when all the problems have been appropriately handled, and when a good plan of follow-up management of the seizures and other problems is developed, the patient is ready to go home.

LEVELS OF DIAGNOSTIC STUDIES

A basic evaluation includes a good examination, blood and urine tests, a brainwave test, and usually x-rays of the head (see Table 7.1). Abnormal findings may indicate the need for further studies, such as an examination of the spinal fluid or a brain scan. Unless the patient is quite ill, or he requires sedation for the test, or the test requires hospitalization, these studies can be done on an out-patient basis. If the results of the tests show the need for more risky studies, as when a correctable cause of the seizures is suspected, the patient is hospitalized. Such studies include injections of dye into the blood vessels to the brain or of air into the spaces around the brain. These procedures are usually performed by a neurosurgeon.

Table 7.1. Minimum diagnostic recommendations

Basic Diagnostic Tests	
Hematologic Studies	Complete blood count
Urine Studies	Urinalysis
Biochemical Studies	Serum calcium and phosphorus; Fasting blood sugar
Serology	Studies to exclude TB, syphilis
Electrophysiologic Studies	EEG
Radiologic Studies	Skull x-ray; Computed tomogram of brain
Psychologic Studies (Child)	Psychologic, psychometric testing
Additional Studies in Select Cases	
Biochemical Studies	5-hour glucose tolerance test; Amino acid screen (inborn errors)
Genetic Studies	Chromosomal analysis (malformations)
CSF Examination	Infections of the nervous system
Electrophysiologic Studies	Special EEG activation procedures (sleep, telemetry, chemical)
Psychologic Studies	Psycholinguistic evaluation for learning problems
Special Studies	
Electrophysiologic Studies	24-hour video and EEG monitoring; Brain surface and depth EEGs
Radiologic studies	Angiogram or Air Study

Adapted from the *Plan for Nationwide Action on Epilepsy* by the Commission for the Control of Epilepsy and Its Consequences.

BASIC STUDIES

The basic studies usually include: examination of the blood count, urinalysis, blood chemistry analysis, sometimes analysis of the cerebrospinal fluid, a brainwave test, a skull x-ray, and sometimes an echoencephalogram (see Table 7.1).

Blood Count

A complete blood count (CBC) checks the number and appearance of red cells, white cells, platelets, and newly formed red blood cells (reticulocytes or retics); it also distinguishes the different types of white blood cells present. This test helps to suggest the presence and possible causes of an anemia (lack of red blood cells), or to indicate an ongoing infection, irritation, inherited metabolic disturbance, allergic reaction, poisonous process, drug reaction, abnormal breakdown or inhibited production of various blood cells, or even various types of blood cancers. A low platelet count may lead to bleeding. A high reticulocyte count means that the blood is being replaced. Another useful test is to let the blood settle over a set period of time. The rate of settling is called an erythrocyte sedimentation rate (ESR). If it is too rapid, this suggests an inflammation or infection. Special studies can be performed, checking for any potential bleeding abnormalities, especially if a dye study of the blood vessels or an operation is going to be done. Special studies can be made for allergic and immune problems, such as lupus erythematosis or other rheumatoid problems.

Urinalysis and Screen for Inborn Metabolic Disorders

The urine is checked for its color, smell, clarity, and density, its protein, blood, and sugar content, and by microscope for excessive red cells, white pus cells, crystals, or clumps of cells or protein molded into a caste. Abnormalities suggest an infection or inflammatory reaction, an excess of chemicals (such as sugar spilling over into the urine), a drug reaction, leaky or inflamed kidneys, body chemical upsets, or damaged and poorly functioning kidneys. An abnormal urinalysis finding and high blood pressure suggest an abnormal kidney as the cause of the seizure.

A screen for inborn metabolic errors can be performed on the urine by adding various chemicals, such as ferric chloride, or paper strips specially treated to detect various substances. Abnormal color changes suggest a metabolic error, drug, or poison. Follow-up testing for further identification can be performed on the blood and on the urine.

Blood Chemistries

Various blood chemicals often should be checked, especially in the acute seizure problem or in the neonate. It is wise to check the blood sugar levels (especially before the patient eats), and often the calcium and magnesium levels. Low levels can cause seizures. If a spot test of the sugar is abnormal, a prolonged 5-hour glucose tolerance test may indicate any blood sugar disorders.

Problems in liver or kidney function can be checked by measuring how these organs handle certain chemicals. An increase in these substances suggests that the organ is not functioning well. It is usually wise to check these functions before starting a new anticonvulsant drug. Periodically rechecking these functions thereafter may be useful.

Special blood studies can be performed if the screening indicates the possibility of an inborn metabolic error, a poison, a drug, a breathing disturbance, or the presence of disease.

Infections and Inflammations

The blood can be checked for specific antibodies that the body has produced to fight off syphilis, viral diseases, or infections before birth. The skull x-ray may show calcium densities from prenatal infections. A skin test for tuberculosis is advisable. In an acute infection a culture and smear to be checked for an infectious agent can be obtained from any body fluid or wound.

Spinal Fluid Examination

A lumbar puncture (LP), performed by inserting a needle between two vertebrae in the lower part of the spine below the end of the spinal cord, is indicated if there is concern about an infection, bleeding, or a degenerative disease of the nervous system. The cerebrospinal fluid (CSF) can be examined for abnormalities, such as an excess of red blood cells (with bleeding), an excess of white blood cells (as with an infection or inflammation), an excess of protein (as with breakdown of a past bleed or of brain tissue), or an abnormally low sugar content (as with meningitis, some tumors, or low blood sugar). A LP should not be done if there is increased pressure within the head unless it is absolutely necessary, and then it must be done very cautiously. It should not be done if there is an infection where the needle would be placed. An LP usually is performed in an acute period of seizure onset when an infection or bleed is suspected or if an ongoing seizure problem is becoming worse.

Special tests may be performed if special problems are to be considered. Just as with blood tests and urinalysis, cultures and smears in search of infective agents and antibodies against these agents can be obtained. If a demyelinative problem is suspected (i.e., the coverings to the nerves are degenerating), a special test called protein electrophoresis may show an elevation of the gamma factors. The CSF can be concentrated and examined under a microscope for abnormal cells, as are seen in tumors.

The EEG (Brainwave Test)

The brainwave tracing or electroencephalogram (EEG) is a method of recording the brainwaves from various parts of the brain. This electrical-chemical energy from the brain portions is picked up by sensitive wires pasted to specific areas on the head. At least 20 such wire leads are used, usually placed in pairs. Since the brain gives off many rhythms simultaneously, the resultant varying energy measurements are transmitted from the leads to a very sensitive machine, the electroencephalograph, which translates these energies into impulses that drive an inkpen stylus. By choice, the technician can direct the energy from one active lead, or from two active leads being compared, to each pen stylus. Depending on the size of the machine, simultaneous recordings can be obtained using 8 or 16 stylus tracings at the same time. This allows tracings from multiple areas of the brain to be recorded at the same time and thus compared. Usually the technician chooses predetermined combinations of leads to be recorded.

As the impulses move the pen tips up and down at various rhythms, a long strip of paper is pulled beneath. This results in 8 or 16 continuous tracing lines on a page, at a rate of about 10 seconds per page. (The average EEG consists of around 12 standard combinations of leads, and usually runs about 500 pages total.) When a sudden energy discharge occurs in the brain, the stylus gives a sudden jerk and then returns to normal; if the discharge is slower, the pen deviation may be a rolling rise and return. Sudden jerks are called spikes because of their sharp points, slower deviations are called waves because of their rolling appearance.

An abnormal brain discharge may cause an abnormal EEG mark, such as a spike or a wave. If the patient has no symptoms, an abnormal discharge is considered an irritation but not a seizure. A seizure is a clinical symptom, not an electroencephalographic finding. However, if the abnormal discharge involves a larger area of the brain or persists for a longer time, the patient may experience symptoms that would be considered a seizure with an EEG confirmation. Not all seizures are confirmed on an EEG. The discharge may come from areas of the brain folded underneath and not near enough to the surface electrodes to be recorded. This is especially true with psychomotor seizures. Sometimes the discharge does not happen frequently enough to be caught during the brief period of time that the EEG is being recorded. Sometimes the typical findings are present only when a patient has a seizure.

To bring out such seizure discharges, special electrodes may be placed, special techniques, such as deep breathing, flashing lights, or sleep, may be tried, or a tracing may be repeated. If the seizure symptoms begin in a foot, special vertex electrodes placed on the top of the head may record the abnormality. Staring spells tend to be brought out by deep breathing, photosensitivity (light-produced) seizures by flashing lights, and psychomotor seizures by drowsiness or light sleep.

Value The EEG can help localize a brain disturbance, help confirm or question a seizure diagnosis, suggest possible conditions that may bring on the seizures, or suggest the possibility of increased risks for a seizure if drugs such as stimulants, tranquilizers, or some sedatives are being considered for use. A series of tracings over a period of time may tell whether the problem is stable, improving, or worsening.

No test is completely reliable. Under the best of conditions, a complete EEG study is only 80% to 90% reliable. If a tracing is obtained only when the patient is awake, less than half of the temporal lobe seizures may be confirmed. Omission of other tests that might bring out seizure abnormalities suggested by the history reduces the accuracy. A tracing is only as valuable as the information given to the technician and her efforts to bring out the suspected discharges.

The value of the EEG is often overestimated. It may locate the seizure discharge but it does not tell what kind of seizures the patient has, what medicine to use, how the patient is responding to the medicine, or when the medicine should be discontinued or changed. It can localize a problem but it does not tell what the problem is or how long it has been there. It does not reveal the patient's age, sex, race, intelligence, learning skills, emotional state, or behaviors. Sometimes, however, it gives hints that can be confirmed or excluded by further examination of the patient.

The tracing is very sensitive. Eye movements, muscle flicks of the forehead, breathing, blood vessel pulsations, the heartbeat, chewing, swallowing, touching a wire, or movements in the room may produce waves that resemble abnormal brain discharges. The EEG machine itself can produce similar artifacts. The technician must distinguish true brain activity from such artifacts. Sometimes the artifact may suggest possible causes for the symptoms, such as an area of excessive muscle artifact with a headache, or an irregular heartbeat artifact. Placing monitoring leads may help to distinguish artifact from seizure fragments in newborn infants.

The Best Tracing Time The ideal time to have an EEG going is when a seizure occurs. This rarely happens. The next best time is at least three weeks after a seizure has occurred, unless the attacks are frequent. An EEG obtained soon after an attack shows the effects of the attack but it may not show the abnormality. It is not as valid as the later tracing. However, a tracing obtained during the hospitalization for the initial attack may show enough to guide further investigations and to help explain the problem to the parents; it can be reassuring even though a follow-up tracing may be necessary.

When ordering an EEG, give a brief history, including a description of the seizures and any abnormal findings on the examination, including skull defects. Note all drugs that the patient is taking, the state of alertness, and any stimuli that might bring on the seizures, so that the technician can use the information to attempt to reproduce such a situation.

Never stop the anticonvulsants for the EEG. The risks of causing a major seizure are too high. There are no therapeutic benefits derived from the EEG. Staying up late the night before may help the patient fall asleep for a more complete tracing, especially if he is anxious. Caffeine-containing drinks (tea, coffee, cocoa, Coke) should be avoided the day of the test. Eating a meal before the EEG helps the patient fall asleep. Often a sedative is given to help the patient relax and sleep.

In addition to the attempt to sleep, designed to bring out psychomotor seizures and additional seizure foci, deep breathing and flashing lights are other common adjuncts to an EEG. If these stimuli produce abnormal, seizure-like bursts on the EEG, they are abruptly stopped before an actual seizure occurs, then retried to confirm that there is a definite, not a chance, relationship between the stimulus and the abnormal bursts. Flashing light is performed at various rates. Sometimes various color filters or specific visual patterns are used to test for special sensitivities.

Special EEG studies can be used, if necessary, on difficult seizure problems. A portable EEG transmitting device can be attached to the patient. While he wanders around a ward at his usual daily ward activities, the transmitted brainwaves are being recorded at the main receiving electroencephalograph. Any observed abnormal behaviors then can be checked to see if they are accompanied by abnormal brainwaves. It is especially useful to have television cameras recording these observations so that the tapes and EEG tracings can be compared later. This is one method by which seizures and behavioral outbursts, e.g., rage reactions, have been differentiated, since the latter produce no abnormal EEG activity.

In patients with uncontrollable focal seizures who may benefit from surgery, special EEG tracings may be obtained. An opening in the skull is made. EEG tracings can be recorded directly from the surface of the brain or from wires sunk deep into the brain. This procedure helps to localize in three dimensions the extent of the abnormal area that is causing the seizures, should the surgeon wish to remove it.

Normal Brainwaves The brain gives off numerous waves at various frequencies in various areas at the same time, with slower waves in the sides, the dominant alpha waves in the back, and faster waves in the front. The overall EEG is much slower in the young child but increases toward normal frequencies by adolescence. Sometimes the posterior head slow waves seen in adolescents and pre-adolescents are mistaken for abnormalities by a person not familiar with children's EEGs.

The EEG changes with falling asleep. New waves begin to appear that indicate when sleep occurs and how deeply asleep the patient is. Common benign findings, such as the so-called 14 and 6 positive spiking phenomenon of childhood, may be seen. This phenomenon was once thought to be a type of behavioral seizure with vague symptoms but now it is felt to be an interesting variant without known clinical symptoms. Even the abnormal findings, as well as the normal frequencies, tend to slow and change their appearance with sleep.

Abnormal Brainwaves In general the brain reacts to an irritant with the break-up of normal rhythms and the appearance of abnormal rhythms. Significant abnormalities, as seen in seizures, include combinations of sharp waves and spikes and slowing of the basic rhythms. These disturbed rhythms are called dysrhythmias. If an insult is more severe, as with actual damage or marked inhibition of brain function, the term used is that of a "delta abnormality," because the faster components disappear, to be replaced by slow, and sometimes high, irregular waves. With a more severe depression of the brain, the brainwaves fade away, taking on a very slow and very low appearance. This is a suppression. If the suppression is very severe, it is sometimes known as a flat EEG, especially when no brain functions can be recorded even though the sensitivity is increased to its maximum and strong stimuli are used. Such a tracing involving the entire brain is usually seen with brain death.

An abnormality may be localized to one part of the brain, to one side of the brain, to several parts of the brain, or to the entire brain. Localized disturbances tend to be more serious than generalized abnormalities. When the two brain halves are not identical either in the rhythm or in the size, the term asynchrony or asymmetry may be used. Consequently the abnormality is described by the disturbance (dysrhythmia, delta, suppression, etc.), the location, and the severity. A grading system is usually used, with grade 1 meaning a mild disturbance and grade 3 meaning a marked and always significant disturbance.

A significant dysrhythmia still bears a rhythmic appearance that may respond to external stimuli and to drowsiness. In seizures such a dysrhythmia may appear as spikes, spike and wave combinations, or multiple spike bursts.

A spike, produced by a sudden discharge of a cluster of cells, usually indicates an irritation to the brain. This abrupt, sharp deviation and return of the pen tip may be followed by a slower deviation, the wave, when the brain is attempting to regain control. The spike can be limited to a small area of the brain, to a large area, or to the whole brain. It may appear as a single spike, a small cluster, or as a series of spikes in a row. It may remain localized or it may spread to other areas of the brain or to the other side of the brain. When the spike spreads to a similar area on the other side of the brain, the EEG shows two focal spikes occurring simultaneously from similar areas of both brain halves. This mirror focus may initially develop with the first spike appearing slightly before the mirror image; however, there is a tendency, as with temporal lobe seizures, for the mirror image to become established and sometimes to break away as an independently firing area. Often with focal spikes there may be slowing of the rhythm in the area of the spike.

Spikes may be brought out by drowsiness and light sleep. With deeper sleep the spike broadens out to become a sharpish wave. Hyperventilation and flashing light may also occasionally bring out a spike focus.

Not all spikes are significant. Some spikes, such as the 14 and 6 per second spikes, are interesting common findings of no proven clinical significance; others, such as the small sharp temporal lobe spikes, phantom spike and wave patterns, and the so-called psychomotor variant patterns, may be significant at times or may also be interesting variants. Sometimes with these latter types a clinical trial of a safe anticonvulsant will be the only way of determining whether the finding is significant.

Another common dysrhythmia pattern is a regular spike/wave pattern. Although these spikes and waves may be focal, often they involve the entire brain. A typical spike/wave pattern repeats three times every second in a monotonous appearance. This is the most common pattern seen with typical absence seizures. Variants of this pattern, such as slower spike/wave patterns, with irregular waves and sometimes extra spikes, may be seen with brain damage. Faster atypical spike/wave patterns may appear later in adolescence. Multiple spikes occurring with the waves is another atypical spike/wave pattern. These atypical patterns may be seen with any type of generalized seizures but they most commonly are seen with atypical absence attacks. They are more difficult to control and are more often associated with other handicaps as well as with persistence into or emergence in adulthood. Sometimes these atypical bursts are triggered by a focal spike discharge, which fires downward to trigger the generalized atypical spike/wave pattern. Deep breathing and flashing lights are most apt to bring out spike/wave bursts, although drowsiness also may bring them out.

A third seizure pattern is hypsarrhythmia, which is essentially found in infancy and is usually associated with infantile myoclonic spasms. Not all cases of infantile myoclonic spasms have hypsarrhythmic patterns. The typical pattern consists of a very high amplitude, disorganized jumble of sharp and slow waves with multiple areas of spikes involving the entire brain. At times the entire picture flattens out for a few seconds and then resumes. Sometimes periodic bursts of spikes may be superimposed on the picture. With a typical hypsarrhythmic pattern, the infant with myoclonic spasms may stop having seizures if he is put on steroids, but the poor outlook for retardation remains the same. The child tends to outgrow this seizure pattern, although later in life he may have focal or multifocal seizures.

A burst-suppression EEG, especially if the bursts occur with fairly regular timing, is not a good finding. The bursts may be associated with myoclonic jerks or twitches. This pattern may be seen after a severe brain insult, such as lack of oxygen, or with a degenerative disease of the brain, such as a slow virus infection. The outlook is poor.

There is no type of dysrhythmic pattern that strictly correlates with any specific seizure, although typical 3 per second spike/wave generalized bursts most often are seen with typical absence seizures and hypsarrhythmia with infantile myoclonic spasms. The pattern during an actual seizure may be different from one between seizures. When a seizure is not occurring, the EEG may be normal, or it may show slow bursts or sharp wave activities, or it may show brief fragments of seizure activities, such as isolated or brief clusters or spikes or spikes and waves. In a seizure there tends to be a very brief period of slowing of normal activities followed by the rapid build-up of faster activities and the appearance of the typical dysrhythmic features. Often the seizure movements produce many muscle artifacts. The seizure attack is associated with a prolonged period of spikes or spikes and waves. With a motor seizure, spiking alone tends to be seen with the stiffening (tonic) phase, whereas the intermixture of the spikes and waves appears with the clonic jerking phase. As the seizure begins to taper off, slower activities replace the faster spiking rhythms and the EEG resolves to a slow, low-amplitude appearance that may remain for some time thereafter.

A delta abnormality implies a more severe brain insult. It appears as very slow, irregular rhythms that are not significantly affected by stimulation. It tends to persist, whereas a dysrhythmia is more intermittent. Deltas suggest damage or severe blockage of normal function. Focal deltas are most worrisome because, although they may be the aftereffects of a seizure, they also could represent a tumor, a stroke area, or a skull defect. Follow-up investigation is usually required.

A summary of abnormal EEG findings is given in Table 7.2.

Skull X-Rays

Skull x-rays are usually obtained in all seizure patients. The possible exception is the typical absence patient. The chance of finding something abnormal by x-ray is small, but the finding may be significant. The major findings are of distortions of the skull's shape or continuity, or abnormal densities of the skull itself or within the skull, i.e., of the brain. Chance findings may be an infection of a tooth, a sinus, or the mastoid air spaces behind the ear. Such an infection could trigger seizures. The major concerns for which a head x-ray is taken are trauma, increased intracranial pressure, a tumor, a congenital defect in the skull, an abnormal blood vessel, or a previous infection in the brain that has left calcium scars behind.

Increased pressure shows up by widening the spaces between the skull bones, increasing the fold-markings that can be seen on the inner surface of the skull bones, and pressure enlargement of the small pocket in the base of the skull where the pituitary gland is located, with the adjacent bone distorted and destroyed.

A fracture may show up as a jagged line running across the skull bones like a bolt of lightning. It must not be confused with the normal sutures, which are the spaces where the skull bones meet. If one side of the fracture is pushed inward, there is increased danger that the brain may be irritated. Not all fractures can be detected by x-ray, although taking a picture across the surface where brain swelling occurs, tangential to the skull, may show up some fractures. Fractures of the base of the skull may be missed but they sometimes cause leaks of spinal fluid into the nose or ears or bleeding around the eyes and ears. The fracture shows only that trauma has occurred. It does not indicate trauma to the brain may have happened; a bruise, tear, or bleed in the brain may be located adjacent to the trauma, opposite it, or elsewhere at places where the brain rebounded or rubbed due to the impact. An analogy to brain trauma can be drawn by visualizing a glass jar, representing the skull, and an egg, representing the brain, within the jar. Hitting the jar with a knife handle may crack or smash the jar without disturbing the egg, unless a chunk of glass digs into it. If instead the jar

Learning About Epilepsy

Table 7.2. Abnormal EEG findings summarized

Name	Meaning	Significance
Artifact	Abnormalities on the EEG tracing that originate elsewhere than the brain	May localize or suggest other causes for the symptoms
Dysrhythmia	Semi-regular, disturbed brain rhythms often responsive to various stimuli	Suggests and locates an irritation to the brain

Spikes
  Sharp Waves,
  Spike/Wave
	Specific types of dysrhythmias of a more significant nature	Suggests and localizes an irritation to the brain; seen with seizures

Hypsarrhythmia	A very high-amplitude disorganized tracing with multiple areas of spikes and sharp waves and periodic generalized flattening	A kind of pattern seen in infants who have myoclonic spasms
Slow Activity	Slower rhythms than expected for the age	Seen with insults inhibiting blood function, after a seizure, in the area of a seizure focus, or with damage
Fast Activity	Faster rhythms than expected at the age	Often seen with irritation or medications or drugs
Burst-Suppression	Low-amplitude to flat picture periodically interrupted by bursts of sharp wave activity	A significant insult or damage, often with significant aftereffects
Normal Variant (14 & 6, etc.)	Specific dysrhythmic patterns commonly found in people	No well-documented correlation to any specific problems
Delta Abnormality	Slow, irregular, and independent activity usually from a focal part of the brain	Severe inhibition or damage as seen with a mass, a stroke, or after a seizure
Asymmetry or Asynchrony	A significant difference in size or rate of the brainwaves between the brain halves	Suggests disturbance on or in one of the brain halves
Suppression	A marked slowing and flattening of the brainwaves	A severe and potentially fatal degree of brain cell inhibition, damage or death

is given a vigorous shake, it may remain intact, but the egg may be smashed. The same principles apply to the skull and brain. Thus the skull x-ray does not tell where or whether any brain damage has occurred.

The skull may be asymmetrical. If part of the brain is damaged or underdeveloped early in life, it will not grow as rapidly. The skull may be flattened in that area and the floor of the skull may be elevated. Asymmetric skulls can be caused by the fusing together at too early a time of two adjacent bones. This may be a primary problem or it may be due to a lack of growth of the underlying brain, which thus allows the bones to close and grow together. If the problem is a primary fusion, it appears very early, with the fusion ridging along the edges of the two bones, and with other parts of the skull overgrowing to compensate. If there is an underlying tumor mass, collection of blood, or enlarged ventricle beneath a part of the skull, that bone area may be bulged out, thinned out, or occasionally thicker and denser.

Abnormal flecks of dense calcium may be seen in the brain with infections around the time of the birth period, with a vascular problem, or with a tumor. The pattern may suggest the cause.

Echoencephalogram (Sonar Encephalogram, Ultrasound Studies)

A safe, quick screening technique especially useful with temporal lobe seizures and after head trauma is the echoencephalogram. An extremely high-frequency sound wave, like a sonar, is passed through from one side of the head to the other and then back again. These sound waves, far above the range of hearing, tend to echo back from any surfaces they hit as they pass through the head. The resultant echoes are measured as blips on a special screen. The usual echoes recorded include a series of echoes from each of the skin-skull-brain surfaces plus a pair of echoes from the third ventricular cavity in the middle of the head. The picture should be symmetrical and the same no matter what the direction of the tracing is. If there is a mass, a lump, a bleed, or a swelling of the brain on the side of the seizure, the midline is pushed to the opposite side. In this case, the midline ventricle echo is shifted away from one side toward the other. If, however, the seizure is associated with brain damage or atrophy (wasting), the shift is toward the seizure side, since there is less brain there. A hint also may be obtained about the ventricular size; for example, in hydrocephalus the midline ventricular echoes are wide apart.

FOLLOW-UP STUDIES

If the preceding studies suggest a potential brain problem, follow-up studies may be needed. These studies often can be obtained without hospitalization unless the patient is quite ill or requires sedation in order to cooperate for a clear picture. These studies include computed tomography, radioisotopic brain scans, and some of the fancier EEG studies previously discussed.

Computed Tomography (CT Scan, CAT Scan, EMI Scan, ACTA Scan)

A safe, new, and major advance in the diagnosis of brain problems is the CT scan. The patient lies on a bed with his head in a circular donut. An x-ray camera is very rapidly rotated within this donut around the patient's head, taking a series of very low radiation x-rays in several planes. This information is fed into a computer, which assembles all the x-ray views at each level and intensifies the small differences in bone and brain density, until the originally hazy picture comes out as a detailed composite picture of one level of the brain. Since a series of planes through the head are studied in this way, the final study appears as a series of computerized pictures at various brain levels. The pictures may be developed in black and white, with various shades of grey representing the various densities, or in color. For example, bone, being very dense, may be white or may be represented by one end of the color spectrum; the brain shows up as various shades of grey or mid-spectrum colors, and the spaces containing CSF, being less dense, show up as dark shades or black, or as a color on the end of the spectrum opposite that of bone. Since the brain consists of structures of varying density, the structures show up as various shades on the final picture.

The CT scan is safe. The radiation is not high enough to be of danger. Often material may be injected into the bloodstream to bring out certain features. Not only does this scan show the shape of the brain and the associated brain cavities and surface, but also, unlike air studies, it can show normal and abnormal structures within the brain. Wasting of the brain surface, ventricular enlargement, or cystic cavities show up as dark areas, whereas solid, dense structures, such as tumors, show up as lighter spots on the picture. Although the study does not make the actual diagnosis of the mass, it may suggest whether the lump seen is hollow, solid and dense, or blood-filled and not too dense. It shows distortions of the brain when they are present.

This study is very useful with seizures. It has a significantly high incidence of abnormal findings, especially with focal seizure disorders. It would be desirable to obtain a CT scan exam on most seizure patients and especially in those with progressive problems, focal disturbances, or abnormal neurologic findings. Yet many of the abnormalities found by CT scan are not treatable, and some clinicians question the value of testing all patients in light of the expense. Careful selection of patients to test may be the best approach.

Isotopic Brain Scan

The isotopic brain scan is a relatively safe procedure, even though it requires the injection of a short-lived radioactive isotope into the bloodstream. As this substance flows through the blood vessels in the head, special counters count the number and location of radioactive emissions given off. The print-outs tend to locate the areas of normal major blood vessels plus any abnormal collections of increased radiation that might suggest an abnormality. Often the study is done in two parts: the first part measures the actual flow of the isotope through the head, and the second part, a few hours later, measures any abnormal collections of the isotope still remaining.

This study is especially useful when abnormal blood vessels, such as malformations, or new blood vessel growth outlining a tumor, an abscess, or a hemorrhage, are suspected. It shows which areas of the brain may be getting a better blood supply and which a poorer blood supply. It also may show areas of increased radiation caused by leaky blood vessels in the area of a malformation or damage. The isotopic brain scan is useful and should be considered when abnormal blood pulsations are heard in the head, when the seizure patient has a vascular red birthmark on his head, when he has pulsatile headaches, or when a brain abscess is suspected. If the flow of blood is blocked to one area of the brain, as in a stroke, the radioactive pickup measured from that part of the brain may be less than normally expected.

FURTHER STUDIES THAT MAY BE RISKY

As the preceding studies identify a possible cause of the seizures, further studies may be necessary if a progressive problem is suspected. These studies usually have a slight risk to them. They should be performed in a hospital with a neurosurgeon at least available, if not actually directing the studies. If problems arise, the patient may need to be taken directly to surgery. These possibly risky studies include angiography, various air studies outlining the nervous system, and the previously mentioned special EEG studies of the brain.

Angiography

Angiography is performed by injecting a dye into the bloodstream. This may be done through a small tube or a fine needle in an artery of the arm, the groin, or the neck. In children it is most desirable to use the groin approach so that the take-off openings of the major blood vessels from the aorta to the head may be seen. A good study includes all the major blood vessels to the brain. The dangers in this study include an allergic reaction to the dye, a bleeding from the vessel, or a spasm or block of the vessel, which can result in a stroke. As the dye flows through the head, a series of x-ray pictures is taken in rapid sequence. This shows the dye-containing blood vessels of the brain. Angiograms are good follow-ups for abnormalities found on an isotopic brain scan. They show abnormalities of the blood vessels, e.g., a malformation, a tumor, a brain abscess, or a bleed. They may help to localize and explain a block to normal blood flow. They may show distortions and displacements from the expected location of various blood vessels, as may be seen with brain swelling, abnormal masses, or hydrocephalus. They show much more detail than the brain scan.

An angiogram probably is not desirable if the patient has a bleeding tendency, irritated or abnormal blood vessels, or a severe kidney disease. Before the study is performed, basic studies should be made to rule out any bleeding disorder and to ensure that the patient has good kidney function. It is wise to have some fresh blood on order should a transfusion be needed.

As a bonus, especially with vascular malformations in children known to have other congenital defects, when the angiogram of the head is completed, the x-ray camera may be shifted down to the abdomen to obtain an x-ray of the dye as it is filtered out through the kidneys and urinary collecting system. Sometimes concurrent x-rays of the heart can be obtained, showing possible malformations and congenital defects.

Air Studies (Pneumoencephalography, Ventriculoencephalography)

The CT scan has largely replaced air studies, since the CT scan, with far less risk, not only shows the outline of the brain that the air studies can show, but also shows structures and disturbances within the brain, which cannot be shown by air diagnostic approaches. In air studies the basic principle is to inject a small amount of air as a replacement for a small amount of CSF. This can be done via a needle inserted into the ventricular system of the brain (ventriculoencephalogram) or through an LP needle in the lower back. The latter is called a pneumoencephalogram. A ventriculogram, rather than a pneumoencephalogram, should be done, even if it means making a surgical defect in the skull, whenever there is the concern about a tumor mass or intracranial pressure. A ventriculogram may be done as the first step in relieving the pressure. A pneumoencephalogram is dangerous with elevated intracranial pressure because the brain could be pushed downward when the fluid is drawn off from below, killing the patient instantly.

With a bubble of air mixed in with the CSF, the patient is turned and tilted at different angles. The various positions cause the air bubble to move around. In each position an x-ray is taken. The sum of all the x-rays should show the outline of all four ventricular cavities plus the brain surface, if the study is complete. Of course no single positioned film shows all the structures; it shows only the areas outlined by the air bubble wherever it has flowed. In contrast, the composite of the views gives the general picture.

If the study is incomplete, showing only a part of the ventricular system, a treatable problem may be missed. The single demonstration of an enlarged ventricle or two, indicative of hydrocephalus, does not explain why the hydrocephalus is present. A complete study may show a tumor that could be surgically removed.

Air studies are good at demonstrating masses in the deep brain, distortions of the shape of the brain, or blocks to the normal flow of CSF throughout the brain cavity system, with resultant hydrocephalus. Wasting or underdevelopment of the brain surface may be shown, although this must be fairly marked to be reliably diagnosed. Many if not all of these findings may be shown as well, if not better, by the CT scan.

Air injection is irritating. It can cause a chemical meningitis or directly irritate the brain and the nerves. It may lead to inflammation and consequent blockage of a marginally functioning CSF flow pathway. It may upset a fragile balance of pressures within the head, resulting in a deterioration of the patient's condition and the need for immediate surgery. A variation of the air study is to inject certain dyes instead of air. These dyes are often more irritating than the air. When an air or dye injection is made, provisions must be made so that the patient can go straight to surgery should any problems arise. If the patient has increased intracranial pressure, the ventriculogram may be the first step in relieving pressure.

Table 7.3 summarizes these diagnostic procedures.

SUPPLEMENTAL STUDIES

The major handicaps of epilepsy are not the seizures; they are the problems of learning and earning and of emotions and behavior. Consequently, evaluations of actual functioning and potential achievement in pertinent learning and employment areas, as well as a survey of emotional stability, can be very helpful to the patient. Such testing should at least be considered in adults; it probably should be a part of the basic evaluation of childhood seizure problems, in light of the high frequency of behavioral complications. The type of testing and the approaches used depend on the age of the child, his needs, and the available resources. The type of seizure, the medications used, and problems noted during a good evaluation may indicate specific needs. An evaluation that omits measurement of functioning in these areas is incomplete.

Testing does not mean just obtaining a cluster of scores; it should include observations of the methods the patient uses in performing the tests as well as the various emotional behaviors he exhibits during the testing sessions. A well-trained evaluator may note evidence of drug reactions or episodes of unsuspected seizure activity; she may even be able to differentiate seizure types and aid the physician in correcting previous diagnoses.

Tests

A variety of tests are available, covering eight major areas of concern: 1) developmental achievement, 2) social maturation, 3) speech and language, 4) general intelligence, 5) educational skills, 6) language and learning processes, 7) vocational aptitude, and 8) prediction of possible emotional prob-

Table 7.3. Diagnostic procedures summarized

Name	Description	Shows
\multicolumn{3}{c}{NON-INVASIVE STUDIES}		

Primary Tests

Name	Description	Shows
Electroencephalogram (EEG)	Very small energy impulses from the brain are recorded by wires pasted to the head and traced out on a long strip of paper as brainwaves	Abnormal electrical activity of the brain, i.e., too much or too little or disordered; also, locates problem
Skull x-ray	X-rays are passed through the head and recorded on photographic film	Shows distortions or erosions of the skull or abnormal densities inside the skull

Secondary Tests

Name	Description	Shows
Echoencephalogram (ECHO, Sonogram)	A very high frequency sound is passed through the head in both directions; the echoes from various structures are photographed and measured	Shows shifts of the brain toward or away from an abnormal EEG area; hints at the size of the midline ventricles
Computed Tomography (CT Scan, CAT Scan, etc.)	A series of low-radiation x-rays are taken by a camera rotated around the head at different levels; the faint results are intensified by computers so that differences in density are clear	Shows distortions, masses, or wasting of the skull, the brain, or the brain surface

lems. With all of these tests it must be remembered that the results are only the means of observing the patient's functioning on the testing day and comparing it to what others his age are expected to be able to do. The score is neither infallible nor a totally reliable label; it is a number value. Illness, overmedication, seizure breakthrough, discouragement, sleep loss, and many other factors may lower the test scores.

Developmental Tests Developmental tests are especially useful in the infant and preschool years. These tests compare movement (both fine finger and gross limb coordination skills), speech and language, social interactions, and adaptive behavior of a child to the average child of the same age. The Denver Developmental Screening Test, the Bayley Infant Maturation Scales, and the Gesell Developmental Skills Inventory are among the more useful developmental tests.

Social Maturation How the child is developing in social skills can be evaluated by tests like the Vineland Test of Social Intelligence, which cover such areas as self-help, self-care skills, social interactions, movements from

Table 7.3 — *continued*

Name	Description	Shows
\multicolumn{3}{c}{INVASIVE, THUS MORE DANGEROUS STUDIES}		
Radioactive Brain Scan	A short-lived radio-substance is injected into a vein; the detector measures the radioactivity as the isotope flows through the brain blood vessels	Shows abnormal collections of blood vessels or leaks of fluid from the blood vessels
Tertiary Tests (If surgery may be needed)		
Angiogram	Opaque dye is injected into blood vessels leading to the head; a series of x-rays is taken as the dye flows through the brain's blood vessels	Shows any distortions, abnormal collections, enlargements, or leakages of brain blood vessels

Air Studies
  VEG = Ventriculogram
  PEG = Pneumoencephalogram
	Air is injected in place of the CSF around the brain, either through an opening in the skull (VEG), or through a needle in the spine (PEG); a series of x-rays is then taken as the air is moved about by tilting the patient in different positions	Shows the shape of the brain and the flow of CSF and air from the ventricles and around the brain

place to place, abilities to communicate thoughts and ideas, and occupational potential. Parents can either overestimate or downgrade their responses. Often a child's measured developmental level reflects his parents' management abilities as much as it measures the child's development.

Speech and Language Some children with seizures have problems in speech and language development, especially if the seizure comes from the left side of the brain. A child's understanding of what is said to him may be evaluated by the Auditory Discrimination Test of Wepman, the Goldman-Fristoe-Woodcock Tests of Auditory Perception and Discrimination, or the Peabody Picture Vocabulary Test. Expressive speech can be tested by such approaches as the Meachem Verbal Language Scales or by observation of and listening to the child's speech. Pronunciation can be evaluated by the Arizona Test of Articulation Proficiency or other such tests. Grammar and syntax can be checked with tests like the Northwestern Syntax Screening Test. Adult patients may be evaluated by use of various tests for receptive and expressive aphasia.

The child with seizures should be referred for speech and language testing whenever a deviation from normal developmental expectations arises. Referral is especially important if the problem is becoming frustrating to either the child or his family. As part of the referral a hearing test should be performed to be sure that faulty hearing is not the problem. Developing proper speech and language not only may help with later learning but also may avoid teasing and taunts by classmates.

General Intelligence There are numerous group and individual intelligence tests, including such screening approaches as the Slossen Intelligence Test. The best IQ tests include the Wechsler intelligence tests and the Stanford-Binet Intelligence Test.

The Stanford-Binet IQ test covers all ages beyond infancy. It tests vocabulary, memory, comprehension, judgment, and problem-solving abilities. However, the IQ score may be depressed in a person with a language or learning disorder, e.g., a person with a left temporal lobe seizure problem.

The Wechsler IQ tests are perhaps more valid and useful psychometric (IQ measurement) test approaches. The Wechsler tests include the Wechsler Adult Intelligence Scale (WAIS), the Wechsler Intelligence Scale for Children (WISC), and the Wechsler Preschool and Primary Scale of Intelligence (WIPPSI). These tests consist of numerous subtests grouped into two major types of learning, verbal intelligence (including general knowledge and the expression of ideas) and performance (including visual motor skills). The individual subtest areas may be useful in developing specific remediation approaches. Specific clusters of subtests may relate to specific types of disturbances or to specific areas of the brain; the overall profile thus may suggest specific problems.

The Cattell Infant Intelligence Scale is more of a test of developmental functioning than it is a predictor of later intellectual potential and achievements.

Intellectual Achievement Tests Educational achievement tests usually evaluate the grade level of achievement in the basic skills of reading, spelling, math, and general knowledge. With reading, for example, a good test not only notes the rate, accuracy, and grade level of performance, it also checks the understanding, recall, and perhaps even the ability to apply the knowledge read. Any academic achievement test should also check the methods used in reading, spelling, and math, since these may need correction or refinement. One of the better tests is the Peabody Individual Achievement Test (PIAT). Another commonly used test is the WRAT. However, the WRAT covers only reading vocabulary recognition, spelling, and arithmetic; it does not check reading abilities and understanding. If the WRAT is used, it must be supplemented by various reading skill tests, e.g., the Durrell Analysis of Reading Difficulty, the Spache Tests of Reading Skills, the Gilmore or Grey Oral Reading Tests, or, with possible learning disabilities, the Slingerland Tests for possible dyslexia. Math problems may be evaluated by such tests as the Key Math Test. There are many other tests used by schools to evaluate performance in these areas.

Psycholinguistic or Neurolinguistic Tests for Learning Disabilities
Specific learning problems are a common finding in children with seizure disorders, especially if the seizures are focal. Children experiencing handicapping difficulties in some but not all areas of schoolwork, those who seem to be struggling along below their potential, or those whose efforts are peculiar or bizarre and significantly below their potential should be referred for learning disability testing. A learning imbalance may exist no matter what the overall intelligence may be. A full learning disability evaluation examines both auditory and visual learning channels, including perceptive recognition, various memory skills, and further learning processes, as well as stages of expression of written, gestured, or spoken thoughts. Such testing should include intelligence and academic achievement tests in order to determine both the general potential and the needs for remediation.

Auditory perception can be tested by using some of the same procedures as in speech testing. Visual perceptual disorders (visuomotor disorders) can be evaluated by tests such as the Frostig Developmental Test of Visual Perception, the Motor Free Visual Perception Test, various Wepman tests of visual perception and memory, the Bender Gestalt Test, the Berea Gestalt Test, the Beery-Buktenica Developmental Test of Visual Motor Integration, and numerous others. Asking the child to copy simple geometric figures or to draw a man may be a useful screening approach.

Further stages of language-learning abilities can be evaluated by a properly performed and interpreted test, such as the Illinois Test of Psycholinguistic Abilities. The Detroit Test of Learning Abilities may occasionally be used with older individuals but it is less specific. A good analysis of the types of errors made in schoolwork, speech, and drawing efforts may give strong indications of problems that the learning disabilities testing then confirms. Specific remediation approaches have been developed to help with specific deficits identified by these tests. However, the remediations are only the beginning. They must be carried over into practical approaches toward improving reading, spelling, writing, math, speech, and coordination. The basic aim is to overcome the problem, get around the problem, or, if nothing else works, to avoid the problem.

Vocational Aptitude Tests Various aptitude tests have been developed for different age groups in order to estimate a person's potential for such activities as schoolwork or future jobs. These evaluations may best be performed in the older child or adult as part of vocational counseling. Vocational aptitude tests may be most important in helping prepare the client for future employment, especially in that the seizure diagnosis may make obtaining a job more difficult. Vocational planning and preparation should not be put off until the patient is past 16 or even in adulthood; it should begin as soon as the diagnosis has been made, with ongoing counseling and guidance as an active part of the seizure management.

Projective Testing for Emotional Problems A good observer and interpreter may gain much information indicating possible emotional problems from the tests described above and from a personal interview with the patient and his family. However, specific testing for emotional problems may be desired, particularly when emotional handicaps are beginning to emerge. The tests may confirm the need for referral for more intensive counseling and guidance. Although the tests are based on objective observations of the performance of thousands of individuals, opinions are mixed about the final interpretations. Some efforts have been made to computerize the test scores. Any interpretation, mechanical or human, that does not take into consideration the effects of the seizures themselves may be tragically in error. Mild seizure bursts, which may be missed by a superficial evaluator, overmedication, or peculiar effects and symptoms of the seizure itself that are honestly reported by the patient all may distort or lower the scores, leading to misdiagnosis if they are not taken into consideration by the interpreter. With temporal lobe seizures the patient may report moments of out-of-contact states, seeing or hearing things, feelings of floating outside of his body, periods of loss of control, episodes of unexplained emotions or recurring thoughts, strange memories, or the feeling that people are trying to control his brain. It is essential that the interpreter realizes that such sensations are typical manifestations of a temporal lobe seizure patient. If he does not realize this, he may mistakenly brand the patient as an early schizophrenic or some other kind of severe psychotic. Beware of overinterpretation.

The Minnesota Multiphasic Personality Test (MMPI) may be an excellent screen for the adolescent or adult patient and for the other family members. It depends on yes/no answers to many questions. The adolescent profile normally is different from the adult profile and the difference must be recognized. If the teenager's profile is that of a normal adult, it suggests that either he has not yet entered into adolescent maturational development or that he has skipped quickly over such development.

Having the patient talk about various pictures may bring out feelings and motives he is otherwise unwilling to talk about. A child may be willing to talk about drawings of a man, a woman, or a house. The individual may be asked to give opinions, express likes and dislikes, answer questions, or make up stories about the pictures (as in a series of cartoons about a dog used in the Blacky Picture Test). He may be asked to express his ideas, feelings, and attitudes about a series of emotionally loaded pictures in the Thematic Apperception Test (TAT) or the Children's Apperception Test (CAT). He may be asked to interpret a series of inkblots, as in the Ror-

Table 7.4. Psychologic evaluations summarized

Peak Age[a]	Indication	Test Type
Preschool +	Developmental delay	Developmental screens
	Social immaturity	Social maturational tests
	Speech and language delays or distortions	Audiometry, Speech and language testing
School-age +	Problems in learning	General intelligence tests
		Academic achievement tests
	School underachievement	Psycholinguistic testing
Adolescent +	Preparation for life	Vocational aptitude tests
	Emotional problems	Projective testing

[a]Whereas the age groupings may indicate the peak age when a problem emerges, some individuals of an older or a younger age may have the same test needs.

schach Inkblot Test, with the evaluator noting the patient's approach to the picture as well as his statements about it. Play therapy using dolls, puppets, or toys may bring out children's feelings.

Another common test is the Sentence Completion Test. The individual is given a series of statements that he is expected to complete. For example, the question might be "The thing that I most like is. . . ." The statements are designed to bring out areas of conflict.

Table 7.4 summarizes commonly used psychologic evaluations by the age groups to which they apply.

Application and Interpretation

The patient must be ready for the test. His seizures should be under reasonable control whenever possible. His medication should be checked to make sure that it is not too strong or giving him side reactions. The patient should be well rested and in good health when he takes the test.

The appropriate tests should be ordered whenever there is a deviation from normal expectations, especially when this becomes frustrating to the parents or handicapping to the child. Such testing should at least be considered and probably screened for whenever the type of seizure or the management approaches place the individual at an increased risk for such problems. In the preschool years, developmental screens, speech and language evaluations, and social development testing may be considered. During the school years, intelligence tests, academic achievement tests, and learning disability testing may become major additional areas. By adolescence, vocational aptitude tests may become an important consideration. At any age, projective testing for emotional difficulties may prove useful.

The test is only as good as the interpreter and the administrator. The purpose of the testing is to document any remediative needs. The remediation must be aimed at overcoming the handicaps identified, not just at improving the test scores. Good testing also should identify strengths that the patient may use to help him develop while he is also trying to catch up in his weak areas. All of these tests are only instruments to evaluate and observe a person's performance in various situations and tasks. The results can be influenced greatly by many factors. The results are not indisputable answers and labels; they are only beginnings. Attitudes, discouragement, and anxiety may significantly distort and depress the testing results. A good testing session and interpretation must consider all of these factors if it is to yield useful and practical results. The evaluator must be the first to question the results if they do not seem to correlate well with the patient's problems. Perhaps he will need to re-evaluate at a later date. The final and best test is the patient's ability to respond to appropriate, practical remediation.

CONCLUSION

The overall purpose of the evaluation is to bridge the gap between the clinical impression and the remediative needs. The diagnostic information, properly interpreted, can be the springboard to an effective management plan. Good seizure care includes not just an evaluation of the seizure proper, but also evaluation and remediation of other problems, especially the consequences of epilepsy.

REFERENCES AND SUGGESTED READING

General

(The) Commission for the Control of Epilepsy and Its Consequences. 1977. Plan for Nationwide Action on Epilepsy. United States Government Printing Office, Washington, D.C. 4 Volumes.
DeMyer, W. 1969. Technique of the Neurologic Examination, 2nd Ed. McGraw-Hill Book Company, New York. 442 pp.
Gomez, M. R., and D. W. Klass. 1972. Seizures and other paroxysmal disorders in infants and children. Current Problems in Pediatrics, Vol. 2, Nos. 6 & 7. Year Book Medical Publishers, Inc., Chicago. 38 pages each.
Lennox, W. G. 1960. Epilepsy and Related Disorders. Little, Brown & Company, Boston. 1168 pp.
Mayo Clinic, Department of Neurology. 1976. Clinical Examinations in Neurology, 4th Ed. W. B. Saunders Company, Philadelphia. 385 pp.
Panfield, W., and H. Jasper. 1954. Epilepsy and the Functional Anatomy of the Human Brain. Little, Brown & Company, Boston. 896 pp.
Singer, H. S., and J. M. Freeman. 1975. Seizures in adolescents. Med. Clin. North Am. 59:1461-1472.
Solomon, G. E., and F. Plum. 1976. Clinical Management of Seizures. W. B. Saunders Company, Philadelphia. 152 pp.

EEG

Aicardi, J., and J. J. Chevrie. 1973. The significance of electroencephalographic paroxysms in children less than 3 years of age. Epilepsia 14:47-55.

Chevrie, J. J., and J. Aicardi. 1972. Childhood epileptic encephalopathy with slow spike-wave. A statistical study. Epilepsia 13:259-271.

EEG-Olofsson, O. 1971. The development of the electroencephalogram in normal children and adolescents from the age of 1 through 21 years. Acta Paediatr. Scand. 208 (Suppl.):7-46.

Foss, A. 1963. Clinical Electroencephalography in Epilepsy and Related Conditions in Children. Charles C Thomas, Springfield, Illinois. 268 pp.

Kiloh, L. G., A. J. McComas, and J. W. Osselton. 1972. Clinical Electroencephalography, Ed. 3. Butterworths, London. 239 pp.

Maheshwari, M. C., and P. M. Jeavons. 1975. The prognostic implications of suppression-burst activity in the EEG in infancy. Epilepsia 16:127-131.

Noriega-Sanches, A., and O. N. Markland. 1976. Clinical and electroencephalographic correlation of independent multifocal spike discharges. Neurology 26: 667-672.

Scott, D. 1976. Understanding EEG, An Introduction to Electroencephalography. J. B. Lippincott Company, Philadelphia. 248 pp.

Tassinari, C. A., G. Terzano, G. Capocchi, B. D. Bernardina, F. Vigevano, O. Daniele, C. Valladier, C. Dravet, and J. Roger. 1977. Seizures during sleep. In: J. K. Penry (ed.), Epilepsy, The Eighth International Symposium, pp. 345-354. Raven Press, New York.

Vanderark, G. D., and L. G. Kempe. 1970. A Primer of Electroencephalography. Hoffman-LaRoche, Inc., Nutley, New Jersey. 48 pp.

Werner, S. S., J. E. Stockard, and R. G. Bickford. 1977. Atlas of Neonatal Electroencephalography. Raven Press, New York. 211 pp.

Computed Tomography

Gastaut, H. 1976. Computerized axial tomography in epilepsy. Epilepsia 17: 337-338.

Gastaut, H., and J. L. Gastaut. 1976. Computerized axial tomography in epilepsy. Epilepsia 17:325-336.

Psychological Testing

Carlson, L. A. 1973. The Nexus. Academic Therapy Publications, San Rafael, California. 160 pp.

Reitan, R. M. 1974. Psychological testing of epileptic patients. In: O. Magnus and A. M. Lorentz de Haas, The Epilepsies 30:559-575. P. J. Vinker and G. W. Bruyn (eds.), Handbook of Neurology. Elsevier North-Holland Publishing Co., New York.

8
ACUTE SEIZURE MANAGEMENT

Most people panic when they come face to face with a person having a seizure. People want to help but they don't know what to do. They fear that the attack will harm the patient or that the patient may harm others. At times the efforts of well-meaning bystanders prove to be more harmful than helpful. Good seizure management begins with knowing what to do and what not to do.

TYPES OF ACUTE SEIZURE ATTACKS

A seizure may present as only a brief fragment of a more typical seizure attack. An incomplete attack may consist of the warning-aura and no more, which suggests that the seizure problem is nearly controlled. A minor adjustment in the daily medications may be all that is needed to gain complete control.

A simple, brief seizure, lasting usually only 5 to 10 minutes and certainly no more than 20 minutes, is the more common occurrence. Appearance of this kind of seizure means the daily medications need to be altered to gain better control. If the seizure is long or severe, a boost of the anticonvulsant drug levels can be obtained by an injection of phenobarbital into the muscle. This will help prevent recurrence while the adjusted daily dosage is taking effect. With most brief seizures a trip to the emergency room, which can be expensive, is not necessary. Rather, the regular physician can be notified of the seizure occurrence within the next few days so that alterations in the medications can be made.

Seizure attacks that last longer or recur within a short period of time are more risky and require more intensive care. A recurrent seizure is one consisting of at least two or three brief attacks separated by one or more hours. The patient tends to recover between the attacks. An injection of phenobarbital or some other anticonvulsant will commonly boost the blood levels high enough to stop the recurrence. The daily medications then need to be adjusted appropriately.

Prolonged seizures last from 20 to 30 minutes up to as long as several hours. Seizure status (status epilepticus) can last from several hours to days. Attacks of status may consist of brief obvious attacks without recovery of consciousness between each episode. Depending on the nature of the episode, these longer attacks can be exhausting to normal body function. Usually the longer attacks either begin as or become generalized motor convulsions. Generalized motor status is dangerous. Occasionally the attack may remain focal, as with focal motor status (sometimes called "epilepsia partialis continuans") or myoclonic seizure status. These focal episodes are more bothersome than dangerous. The danger of a focal attack is the potential for it to burst forth into a generalized motor status. Prolonged and confusional episodes may be the main symptom of absence and psychomotor status. Control of these attacks usually requires a combination of injections of various anticonvulsants directly into the bloodstream or into the muscle, and then adjustment of the ongoing daily dosages. The patient usually requires significant medical support during these periods. The anticonvulsant is often continued at a stronger than usual dosage for several days after the episode has been controlled in order to guard against recurrence.

DANGERS OF LONG OR FREQUENTLY RECURRING SEIZURES

A long, severe, or frequently recurring seizure is a major stress to the body. The abnormal movements and stiffening interfere with breathing. The excessive amount of secretions and problems in getting rid of them also interfere with breathing. Often the physician who listens to the chest of the patient immediately after the seizure suspects a pneumonia or chest infection because of the rattles he hears, but the noises clear up within hours after the seizure has stopped. However, the patient may choke on these secretions. He may gag and vomit during the attacks, causing further problems with breathing that can lead to his not getting enough air into the lungs and consequently an insufficient amount of oxygen to the brain. The patient may appear blue. If breathing problems are prolonged, the brain and other body organs may be damaged. The brain needs extra oxygen and blood sugar during the energetic discharges of the seizure. If it is not well supplied, brain function falters and may fail.

The body responds in many other ways to a long or hard seizure. Initially the blood pressure rises, the heartbeat increases, and the blood sugar level rises above normal. The excessive activity and use of oxygen and blood sugar leads to an excess of acid in the body. If the seizure continues for a long time, the supply of blood sugar for energy may become exhausted, although the increased need continues. The blood pressure, both because of the exhaustion to the body and due to the high dosages of anticonvulsants being given, tends to fall sometimes to dangerously low levels. The body acidity changes to an alkalinity, which depresses heart and breathing activities. The excessive muscular activity often causes the patient to develop a fever, which at times may become extremely high. The strain on the muscles and their bony attachments may be too much, and muscular strains or tears, as well as fractures of the bones, may occur. The heart and the respiratory system become exhausted by the strains of keeping up with the demands of the long attack.

The drop in blood pressure, the erratic circulation of blood by the blood vessels, some of which constrict and some of which dilate, as well as the interferences with normal breathing, result in an inadequate delivery of oxygen-carrying blood to the brain and an inadequate removal of the waste products from the brain and muscles. The fall in the blood sugar and the fever excesses are additional insults affecting the brain, heart, and respiratory system. These factors can cause death or can result in brain damage. The insult to the brain can result in new seizure problems, a drop in learning and intellectual skills, new neurologic handicaps, or behavioral instabilities. A lengthy seizure can be fatal due to vomiting and inhalation of the vomited materials, accidents resulting from the seizure, brain swelling, or failure of the heart or respiration.

MANAGEMENT OF ACUTE SEIZURES

The goal in acute management should be to control the seizure as quickly as possible without allowing any harm to come to the patient. Failure to achieve or to maintain control within a reasonable time is usually due to an avoidable delay in beginning therapy, too small a dosage of medication, administration of medications by the wrong approach, or failure to maintain control once it has been achieved. Occasionally, failure to control the seizure breakthrough is due to overlooking an infection or an acute irritation.

Basic Care

Remain calm. This may be the first seizure those around the patient have experienced but it may not be the patient's first attack. Common sense should prevail. Remain at the patient's side rather than running for help. Call for aid if it is needed.

Prevent the patient from hurting himself. Lay him on a bed or on the floor or ground. Remove any furniture or objects that he might hit during the convulsive movements. Remain at his side to help with any problems that may arise. Don't attempt to restrain his movements. Although a patient will not purposefully harm anyone during an attack, the uncontrolled, powerful movements are apt to hurt others who get in the way.

Roll the patient onto his side. (Use of the arm and the bended knee as a lever can roll even the heaviest of patients.) This position allows the tongue to fall forward and to the side, allowing more room in the air passage. Don't place a pillow beneath the patient's head; this tends to cramp the breathing passages. Instead, if needed, place the pillow beneath the patient's hips. Tilting him with his head slightly downward helps to drain the excess secretions and vomitus, should the latter occur; it also may help if the blood pressure drops.

Tip the head back and pull the jaw forward. This moves the tongue out of the way of blocking the air passages. If the patient is left on his back, and especially if a pillow is placed beneath his head, bending his head forward, the tongue tends to drop backward, blocking the airway. This problem is what people really mean when they use the term "swallowing his tongue," an act which is anatomically impossible.

Do not stick fingers, padded tongue blades, or hard objects into the mouth in order to protect the patient from biting himself. Usually such an effort is already too late. Fingers can be bitten severely. Other objects can damage or knock out teeth. Damaged teeth may alter the facial appearance adversely and the patient with seizures already has enough of a handicap. Damaged teeth may be more prone to irritate the gums, causing overgrowth when the patient is on Dilantin. The danger of knocking a tooth into the lung, causing a lung abscess, is a serious concern. If there is a need to place anything between the teeth, a soft cloth, folded or twisted, is probably safest and most readily available. The cloth should be inserted gently, never forced. (In medical facilities, sometimes an airway is gently inserted between the teeth to assist in breathing and in suctioning out the secretions.)

Loosen any tight clothing, especially those around the patient's neck. Remove any loose bedding that might cover the patient's face, causing further breathing problems.

If the patient's nails, hands and feet, or face appears bluish, he needs help in breathing. Mouth-to-mouth resuscitation may be needed if simple repositioning does not help. If available, oxygen and use of an Ambu-bag to assist breathing can be most beneficial.

Medical Management

High dosages of anticonvulsants, administered by more direct routes than merely increasing the oral dosage, are necessary to control prolonged seizures. The anticonvulsants most commonly used in acute seizure control are phenobarbital, Valium, Dilantin, and paraldehyde. Other, faster-acting barbiturates (Seconal, Nembutal, Pentothal), other anticonvulsants, such as clonazepam and sodium valproate, or other medications, such as chloral hydrate, lidocaine or procaine, magnesium sulfate, or ether, may occasionally be used.

Valium is a very fast-acting drug. It must be given as an injection into the bloodstream. Its controlling effect occurs within a few minutes. Any bad effects on breathing and blood pressure usually appear within the first 5 minutes and often last only 5 to 10 minutes. Valium may not be totally effective with an acute, ongoing irritation to the brain. It is the best medication to begin with, since it gains the most rapid control and has the shortest danger period. However, the effect of Valium wears off rapidly, lasting only 15 to 45 minutes. Valium may be repeated as needed but it is usually best to use it to get control and then to use another, longer-acting anticonvulsant to maintain control.

Phenobarbital can be given by any route. When used to control a seizure, it is given as a large dosage injected into the bloodstream. When used to maintain control already achieved, it can be given in smaller (hence safer) dosage by injection into the muscle or beneath the skin. Phenobarbital, like Dilantin or paralydehyde, takes as long as 15 to 30 minutes to reach its peak effect. The potential problems in breathing and a drop in blood pressure may appear with the peak; these problems may continue for up to 45 minutes, requiring ongoing support. The effect of phenobarbital, like that of Dilantin or paraldehyde, lasts for at least 4 to 6 hours. These are good drugs to continue control.

Paraldehyde is a strongly odorous medication that can be given by several routes. It can be irritating if it is injected into the muscle or if it is given by a tube inserted into the stomach. It is slowly absorbed if given by a tube into the stomach or as an enema into the rectum. It is very difficult to mix because of its oily consistency, and therefore it is difficult to give directly into the bloodstream; the injection must be given carefully and slowly to prevent inhibition of or irritation to respiratory function. The medicine can decompose, forming poisonous substances, if it is stored in the sunlight. It can react with plastic syringes or plastic tubing, jamming the apparatus or causing poisonous by-products. Paraldehyde, like the faster-acting barbiturates, ether, or chloral hydrate, works primarily by putting the patient to sleep. If handled correctly and given cautiously, it can be a very effective and fairly safe drug. Often it is used by carefully giving divided dosages as shots into the muscle. It is less apt to disturb breathing by this method.

Dilantin, a high-dose injection into the bloodstream, can be most effective. There is some evidence suggesting that too high a dosage may harm the balance and coordination centers of the brain, but so can a prolonged seizure. If given too rapidly, Dilantin can produce irregularities of the heartbeat and a marked agitation. Dilantin should never be given as an intramuscular injection because it rapidly crystalizes. The result is that a rapid blood level rise is not obtained when needed, but, as the crystals slowly break down, the blood levels rise and fall for weeks afterwards.

Methods Methods used in giving the medication are important. Quick control can be achieved only by giving the anticonvulsant into the bloodstream. The main dangers of this route are in causing slowing or stoppage of breathing, a dangerous drop in the blood pressure, or, occasionally, irregularities of the heartbeat, which can happen at the time of the initial injection, especially if the injection is given too rapidly, or, what is more likely, when the drug reaches its peak effect. The medical staff must be on guard against this danger both at the time of the initial injection and at the later and lengthier period when the peak effect of the medication is anticipated. The pulse, breathing, and blood pressure must be checked repeatedly until these danger periods have passed. These risks are especially high if the drugs are given at a high dosage or if multiple anticonvulsants are given over a short period of time. There is an additive risk in the latter situation, especially if the peak effect periods occur simultaneously. Problems have arisen when phenobarbital was given before Valium, rather than after it, because the delayed peak effect of the phenobarbital occurs at the same time as the rapid peaking of the Valium; by first giving the Valium and then the phenobarbital, one separates these danger periods.

Giving an injection into the muscles (except with Dilantin) produces lower blood levels but prolongs the effectiveness of the anticonvulsant. The blood level is usually not great enough to cause any problems unless massive dosages are used. The injections may be irritating to the muscle. This approach is a good method for maintaining control but not for achieving the initial control.

Giving the medication by mouth to stop an ongoing seizure or to prevent recurrence in the acute period is ineffective. In an ongoing seizure there is the danger that the patient will vomit up the medication. Even with a strong dosage, it takes several days to build up an adequate protective level. This is why phenobarbital given only by mouth to prevent a febrile seizure in young children is not effective. The giving of anticonvulsants by an enema or suppository may yield faster but more erratic responses, especially if the patient is due for a bowel movement.

Precautions Precautions must be taken when the anticonvulsant is given in a high dosage, especially if it is injected directly into the bloodstream. The medical staff should be prepared to check blood pressure, pulse, and respiration; they should be prepared to breathe for the patient, with oxygen available, should the respirations slow dangerously. They should be prepared to maintain an adequate blood pressure. Raising the lower end of the bed may help to increase the blood pressure and the blood supply to the brain.

Treatment Treatment of the seizure depends on the type of attack. An attack lasting less than 10 minutes usually requires only an adjustment in the daily medication. A severe, recurrent, or prolonged attack that has resolved by the time the patient is seen by his physician may require an intramuscular boost of an anticonvulsant, such as phenobarbital, and adjustments in the daily medication. An ongoing attack requires a more vigorous approach. An injection of a fast-acting anticonvulsant, such as Valium, into the bloodstream is used. If it doesn't have an effect within 5 to 10 minutes, it may be repeated. If this works, then a longer-acting anticonvulsant, such as phenobarbital, can be injected into the muscle to maintain the control begun by the Valium. The phenobarbital need not be given in the maximum dosage under these circumstances and the giving of the dosage about 10 to 15 minutes after the initial Valium injection prevents many of the potential side effects.

If the seizure does not respond to Valium, a higher dosage of phenobarbital may be given into the bloodstream. The patient must be watched more carefully for acute and delayed heartbeat, blood pressure, and breathing reactions. Should this not work, Dilantin and paraldehyde can be tried. Anticonvulsant injections can be repeated at 20- to 30-minute intervals. If a drug is repeated at such intervals, usually it is safer to use one-half to two-thirds of the maximum initial dosage at the time of the repeat dosage. Waiting this period of time gives the drug a chance to take effect.

If the convulsions continue despite repeated injections of the more common anticonvulsants, more intensive approaches can be used. The patient must be hospitalized and monitored very carefully. Various sedatives, such as the faster-acting barbiturates, chloral hydrate, or inhaled ether, may induce both sleep and seizure cessation. Magnesium sulfate is useful if the cause of seizures is high blood pressure. Sometimes drugs such as lidocaine or procaine, which are local anesthetics that can also be used to control irregular heartbeats, are useful if given by adjustable slow drips into the bloodstream.

Ongoing Support Ongoing support of the patient during the seizure is absolutely necessary. If the patient is having breathing difficulties or is bluish despite good positioning and the active draining and suctioning out of the excessive secretions, assisted breathing is needed to prevent brain damage. If nothing else is available, give mouth-to-mouth resuscitation. An Ambu-bag and oxygen may be needed. An airway may be inserted to assist in keeping the airway open and in suctioning out secretions. Giving oxygen for 5-minute periods at least 3 to 4 times an hour may be most beneficial. Artificial respiratory support may become necessary if high dosages of anticonvulsant medication or the exhaustion of a lengthy seizure leads to respiratory failure.

High blood pressure during a seizure will usually drop as the anticonvulsant medications begin to accumulate, unless the hypertension is the cause of the seizure. If high blood pressure is the cause, additional medications to reduce the blood pressure and overcome spasms in the blood vessels may be necessary. It is desirable to lower the blood pressure fairly rapidly, but not too quickly. If the blood pressure falls more rapidly than the blood vessels in spasm begin to relax, the areas of blood circulation beyond the spasm are apt not to receive enough blood, leading to swelling and damage.

Of more common occurrence is a drop of the blood pressure to dangerously low levels. This can be caused by the anticonvulsant drugs or the exhaustion of a long seizure. Low blood pressure results in an inadequate supply of blood to the brain. Tilting the patient with his head below the level of his hips and legs helps to increase the blood flow to the brain. Medication may be needed to raise the blood pressure to an acceptable level.

A high fever of 103° or more may be the cause or the result of a lengthy seizure. Either way, the fever can be harmful. The temperature should be lowered to 100-101° by active intervention and then it should be allowed to normalize on its own. The patient may be sponged in lukewarm water and then cooled gradually, to prevent shivering, by adding cooler water or even a small amount of alcohol to the bath. Shivering is to be avoided because it causes the fever to go up. Sponging is most effective if the patient is undressed so that as much skin surface as possible is exposed to radiate heat. The skin should be rubbed vigorously with a wet cloth, rotating the rubbings from one part of the body to the next. For extremely high fevers, ice water or ice-packing, or the use of a mechanical cooling blanket, may be necessary. Sometimes chlorpromazine must be given to prevent shivering. These efforts should reduce the fever to below 101° but not all the way to normal. A rapid drop in temperature may be more harmful than helpful if attempts are made to get the fever immediately to normal. Obviously, before these attempts are begun, the patient should be given aspirin or some similar fever-reducing medicine by mouth or by rectal suppository so that it can be taking effect to maintain the temperature control after the more vigorous methods initiate the fever reduction. It takes at least 30 minutes for the medicine to begin to work. Since the aspirin or similar medicines usually hold their effect only about 4 hours, the patient must be watched carefully; he may need a repeat dosage of medicine 4 hours after the original dose.

Often a seizure of one-half hour or more leads to upsets in important blood chemicals, including a drop in the blood sugar and the build-up of acid and alkaline substances in the body. An injection of sodium bicarbonate into the bloodstream may overcome the latter problems, which otherwise might lead to heart and breathing failure. Giving a concentrated injection of sugar into the bloodstream will not hurt the patient and may be most helpful if the blood sugar stores are exhausted. Blood samples to check for possible imbalances should be drawn before corrective injections are given and especially if the patient is to be kept on intravenous fluids for a period of time. The unconscious patient may need such fluid maintenance for a prolonged period. The amount of fluids the patient receives and the amount that he loses via urine, vomiting, etc., must be monitored carefully. It is best to give only about 80% of the anticipated needed fluids. This "drying out" for a brief period of time may help overcome swelling of the brain (edema), a common occurrence with long seizures. Administering concentrated solutions of various sugars, mannitol, or urea, or administering such drugs as Lasix or other medications that pull fluids out of the brain may help to overcome this tendency toward brain swelling. Decadron or other steroids may be given to overcome the brain edema also, although theoretically steroids should not be very effective with this type of swelling.

Continued Control Continued control of the seizures is important. Additional anticonvulsants are usually begun 3 to 4 hours after the initial controlling medications have been given. If the patient has not previously been on an adequate amount of anticonvulsants, a strong dosage (at least twice the usual daily dosage) may be given for the first two to three days. This allows a quicker build-up of a protective body level of the drug. After three days of total seizure control, the medication is reduced to the regular dosage, adjusted to prevent further seizures.

WHY DID THE SEIZURE OCCUR?

Discovering the cause of the attack is most important. With the patient's first attack, this discovery is the goal of the evaluation. With a recurrent attack, it is important to find out what caused the unexpected recurrence, so that the seizure will not happen again.

The most common causes by far of a breakthrough seizure or of a prolonged attack are an infection or the missing or sudden stopping of medication. Medicines may be forgotten occasionally without harm, but forgetting too often can lead to a seizure. Sometimes medications are mistakenly omitted for an evaluation or for an EEG. Sometimes the patient runs out of medications and delays in getting the needed refill. Occasionally the refill of a prescription is not the same as the original dosage. Sometimes the patient or his physician begins to reduce a medication too rapidly. Since problems with taking medication are among the most common causes of a seizure breakthrough, obtaining a blood sample for an anticonvulsant measurement before giving injections of the anticonvulsant may indicate the need for counseling. Skipping medications can be a form of denial of the seizure problem. Sometimes a patient deliberately misses enough medications so that his seizures will not be totally controlled, since, if his seizures were totally controlled, he would no longer qualify for special benefits.

The dosage and the appearance of the medicine that the patient states he is taking should be compared to what was prescribed and what the patient is thought to be taking. Differences may indicate where the error is. If the seizures begin to break through while the patient is in the hospital, checking the hospital chart for the written orders and for the medications actually given may reveal omitted dosages and mistaken orders.

Some children will have a seizure as an early sign of developing infection. With young children and with retarded individuals an unexpected seizure breakthrough may call attention to a hidden infection, such as an ear infection. With some individuals, the seizures will not be controlled well until the infection is controlled.

Other stresses, such as the onset of a menstrual period, sleep irregularities, emotional stresses, alcohol or drug intake, allergies, or an active irritation within the head, will cause a seizure breakthrough. Whenever the cause of the seizure breakthrough is found, be it missed medicines, an infection, an active problem within the head, or some other stress, further care, counseling, and possible alternate or additional management methods may be developed to prevent any future recurrence.

REFERENCES AND SUGGESTED READINGS

Bruya, M. A., and R. H. Bolin. 1976. Epilepsy: A controllable disease. Classification and diagnosis of seizures. Am. J. Nurs. 76:388-397.

Dodson, W. E., A. L. Prensky, D. C. DeVivo, S. Goldring, and P. R. Dodge. 1976. Management of seizure disorders: Selected aspects, Part 1. J. Pediatr. 89:527-540.

Khalid, M. S., and H. Schulz. 1976. The treatment and management of emergency status epilepticus. Epilepsia 17:73-76.

Livingston, S. 1973. Seizure disorders. In: S. S. Gellis and B. Kagen (eds.), Current Pediatric Therapy, Ed. 6, pp. 78-92. W. B. Saunders Company, Philadelphia.

Richens, A. 1976. Drug Treatment of Epilepsy. Year Book Medical Publishers, Inc., Chicago. 176 pp.

Scholl, M. L. 1966. Epilepsy in Children. In: H. F. Conn (ed.), Current Therapy, pp. 574-581. W. B. Saunders Company, Philadelphia.

9
ONGOING ANTICONVULSANT MANAGEMENT

The goals of good seizure management, in order of descending priority, are: 1) to help the patient achieve the best functioning he has potential for; 2) to try to control the most bothersome seizures (e.g., major seizures and drop attacks are more handicapping than absence attacks); 3) always to keep trying to control all seizures, even though this may seem an impossible task. Some physicians mistakenly reverse these priorities, putting complete seizure control as their main objective and sacrificing the patient's alertness and coordination. These physicians fail to realize that a person with an occasional seizure may lose up to an hour or so out of a day because of a seizure, but a person who is overmedicated in an effort to control all seizures loses his whole day, since his thinking and performance are slowed by the drugs.

The total approach in seizure management is aimed at 1) seizure control, 2) helping with the consequences of epilepsy, and 3) counseling the patient and his family about present problems and potential difficulties. Drug management can be thought of in five stages: 1) beginning medication, 2) adjusting dosages, 3) adding further medication, 4) transferring from one drug to another, and 5) discontinuing anticonvulsant therapy.

BEGINNING THERAPY

There is a high risk for recurrence of a seizure if a patient is not placed on protective anticonvulsant medication. This chance is much smaller once therapy is begun. Indeed the chances are quite good that the seizure disorder can be controlled, especially if the control is achieved and maintained within the first three to six months of good therapy. Yet not all patients need be rushed into treatment, especially if a seizure is suspected but not con-

Table 9.1 Specific medicines for specific seizures

Seizure Type	Barbiturates	Dilantin	Tegretol	Minor Medications
Generalized Motor / Psychomotor / Focal	+ + +	+ + +	+ + +	±
Atypical Absence / Akinetic / Myoclonic	+	+	+	+ + +
Typical Absence	−	−	0	+ + +
Mixed Seizures	+ +	±	+	±
Toxicity Rating	+	+ +	+ + +	+ + +

firmed. Unless the EEG is definitely abnormal, it may be better to wait to observe further spells so that a better description of the attacks can be obtained. However, if the EEG is definitely abnormal, one of the safer anticonvulsants may be tried to see if it produces a significantly beneficial effect. If a patient experiences a single, brief seizure without an obvious cause, some physicians would begin treatment only if the EEG is abnormal. Otherwise they would wait until the seizure recurs. Other physicians would treat the first definite seizure regardless of the EEG findings, although they would prefer EEG confirmation. Nearly all physicians would begin therapy if the first seizure was long or severe or if the seizures recur.

Types of Anticonvulsants

There are essentially only four groups of anticonvulsant drugs, 1) the barbiturates, 2) the hydantoins, such as Dilantin, 3) the iminostilbene chemicals, such as Tegretol, and 4) a miscellaneous cluster of related chemical families useful in treating the minor seizures, e.g., the absence, akinetic, and myoclonic attacks. These may be called the "minor seizure medications."

Table 9.1 lists the specific seizure disorders for which these four groups of drugs are used. Each group is discussed in detail below.

The barbiturates, including phenobarbital, its weaker cousins Mebaral and Gemonil, and a stronger relative, Mysoline, are a relatively safe and cheap group of drugs that can suppress a focal discharge, prevent the spread of the seizure from the abnormal focus throughout the brain, and enhance the overall seizure inhibition tendencies of the brain.

The principle hydantoin in use is Dilantin. Although it has no significant effect on the seizure focus, it is most powerful in preventing the spread down the nerve pathways of the brain, but in a different manner than the barbiturates do. It may aggravate the tendency toward typical absence seizures and have variable effects on the atypical forms. Dilantin has many more bothersome and risky side effects than the barbiturates.

Tegretol, the only iminostilbene chemical now actively used for seizures, is a new drug. It appears to be a very effective drug with fewer sedative effects; indeed, it may be especially useful for patients with behavioral problems. Its increased risks and remaining Federal drug restrictions have limited its usage. The barbiturates, Dilantin, and Tegretol are most useful in treating the generalized motor seizures, focal seizures, and complex psychomotor seizures. They may have some beneficial effects with other seizures, except for the typical absence attacks, which may be increased.

The "minor seizure medications" consist of several similar chemical families: 1) the succinimides (Zarontin, Celontin, Milontin), 2) the oxalodiones (Tridione, Paradione), 3) the benzodiazepines (Valium, Clonipin), 4) a new drug, Sodium Valproate, and 5) a weak anticonvulsant, Diamox. For typical absences, Zarontin, Tridione, Clonipin, and possibly Valproate are especially beneficial. For the atypical absence, akinetic, and myoclonic attacks, Clonipin, Valium, and Valproate are the most effective. Celontin is a drug to consider in mixed seizure disorders, such as atypical absence and psychomotor attacks. Valproate may also be effective. In general, these drugs are slightly more risky than Dilantin. Consequently, they must be monitored more closely.

Approach

One Drug at a Time Always begin only one drug at a time. Beginning multiple drugs simultaneously not only may lead to confusion should a seizure occur, but also subjects the patients to the inconvenience and risks of taking drugs that might not be needed, as well as possibly aggravating the seizure problem. Initially, a single drug should be selected that will most likely control the seizure yet cause the least bothersome or risky side effects. Phenobarbital is probably the safest, the cheapest, the most effective, and thus the best drug to begin with, no matter what the seizure type is. Some physicians prefer to begin with Dilantin; however, the risk of side effects is much greater with this drug. Also, the common cosmetic side effects of Dilantin may be more disturbing to the adolescent girl than are the seizures. Children may have increased difficulties with gum overgrowth. A woman in or nearing her childbearing years may have a deformed baby because of the Dilantin. Thus there are numerous disadvantages but no proven advantages in beginning with Dilantin. Moreover, in a preschool-age child, and especially in infancy, the erratic absorption of Dilantin makes the adjustment of a stable blood level difficult, especially since a younger child is less likely to display the early signs of intoxication.

If a child presents with typical absence seizures only, some physicians prefer to begin with Zarontin or some other minor medication. However, such a patient is also at risk for developing a major seizure attack and this tendency may be aggravated by the "minor medication." Many physicians will begin with phenobarbital to protect against the major attacks. Occasionally phenobarbital used alone may control the seizures, but more often it increases the frequency of the minor attacks. If the staring spells continue after three or four weeks of phenobarbital, Zarontin is then added to the therapy.

Dosage and Form Usually the patient is begun on the average dose for his age. Sometimes a low dose is begun and gradually built up in stages every 4 to 7 days over a 3- to 4-week period. This method can avoid some early side effects, and is used most frequently with Mysoline, Clonipin, and Tegretol, although it may be used with the other drugs, especially if the child is in school. In general, the rule is that the infant and, to a lesser extent, the preschool child require a higher dose per unit of body weight and more frequent administration of the drug during the day, a phenomenon that is related to the faster body metabolism and consequent drug turnover in the younger child. At around 8 to 10 years of age the dose calculation changes over from a weight-based dose to a low adult daily dose. The 10- to 12-year-old may take about two-thirds of an average adult dose.

It is far more desirable to prescribe the anticonvulsant as a tablet than as a liquid. It is nearly impossible to keep a suspension evenly mixed, despite vigorous shaking. Liquids are less accurately measured, more likely to be spilled, spit out, or drooled during the administration, and are less absorbable, more expensive, and more difficult to pick up if the container is broken. As soon as the infant is able to eat semi-solid foods, he can take tablets crushed and hidden in a spoonful of acceptable food. Capsules also may be emptied into food. Some capsules contain liquid, which may be squeezed into a more strongly flavored liquid. Sometimes these liquid capsules can be given in half strength by freezing the capsule and then cutting it in half, mashing the frozen contents into food. Some medications may require strongly flavored foods to cover up their bitter taste.

Frequency and Time The number of times the medicine must be given during the day depends on the rate of turnover of the drug in the body and the age of the child. Drugs with a slow rate of turnover, like phenobarbital, Dilantin, Mebaral, and perhaps Zarontin, may be given only once or twice a day in the adult and yet still maintain an adequate blood level. However, the risk in this procedure is that, if the patient forgets a dose, he forgets his entire day's medication, which might be a major omission. Furthermore, a single dose of Dilantin may be irritating to the stomach; it might be less irritating to give Dilantin at least twice a day. Because of the more rapid metabolism of the younger child, he may need to be given Dilantin two to three times a day; the infant may need a dose three or four times a day for the same reason.

Tridione probably needs to be given two or three times a day. Drugs like Celontin, Valium, Clonipin, Tegretol, Diamox, and Mysoline have a fairly rapid turnover, and often are best given three or four times a day.

Mysoline is a special type of drug. It breaks down into two major anticonvulsants, a fast-acting form, abbreviated PEMA, and a slow-acting component, phenobarbital. To maintain adequate blood levels of each of its components, Mysoline may best be given as two or three smaller doses during the daytime and a larger dose at bedtime.

Giving medicines along with meals tends to reduce the absorption of the drug; however, a meal reduces the tendency of some drugs to irritate the stomach and serves as a strong reminder to take the medication. Whenever possible, it is desirable to avoid a child's having to take medication during school hours. Often this can be accomplished by scheduling medication at breakfast time and at suppertime or after school, with a third, larger dose at bedtime. However, some children may also require a noontime dosage in order to control their seizures, and this dosage can easily be administered by the school nurse or the child's teacher.

If the heaviest dosage of the medicine is given at bedtime, an adequate blood level is maintained, affording protection throughout the night, when seizures are most likely to occur, yet the slight intoxication effects are covered by the sleep. This nighttime protection is often a relief to the parents. Further adjustments in the medicines depend on the timing of the seizure breakthroughs and of any side effects.

Prescriptions Frequently Federal law requires that prescriptions for certain drugs, including some of the anticonvulsants, be given for only one month at a time, with a renewal monthly for up to a six-month period. Although these restrictions on prescribing larger quantities of certain drugs result in a slightly higher cost, it is probably wise not to have more than a month's supply of pills available at any one time, especially if the patient's family includes small children who might get into the containers. The family or patient should be sure to contact the physician for a prescription as soon as the last refill has been obtained, since it is dangerous to run out of medication and risk a breakthrough seizure. Often the need for a new prescription correlates with the need for the patient to be seen again.

The patient and his family should be very familiar with the appearance (form, color, shape, markings) and strength of the medicine, and with any numbers or letters marked on each medicine. This knowledge will help safeguard against errors in refilling the medicine. Also, a card listing each medication, including the strength and the dose schedule per day, should be carried in the patient's purse or billfold; if the patient is involved in an accident and is unconscious, the emergency room personnel can use the information on the card to manage his anticonvulsant needs. Although engraving information about medication on a bracelet or necklace is an effective idea with other conditions, many epileptic patients experience enough changes in their anticonvulsants that this probably is not a practical approach for them.

Involvement of the Patient and Family   It is necessary that the adult or child and his family be informed not only about the seizure and related problems but also about the medicines that will be prescribed. This information should include a discussion of the purpose of the drug, its expected benefits, and its more common side effects. Depending on his age and intelligence, the patient should assume as much responsibility as is reasonable for taking his medications. To get him to do this, the medical staff must convince him that the medicine is needed.

The patient, the family, and the school should be encouraged to contact the physician should any possible side effect be suspected. Discovering a side reaction early, before it becomes severe, may reduce the danger and difficulty in handling the problem. Similarly, the physician should be informed of an unexpected seizure breakthrough soon after its occurrence, not months later. A good physician checks out any problems and makes all possible adjustments to avoid any further problems.

The physician should be readily available to the patient and family and he should encourage questions about the seizures and the medications. An open and free interchange may reveal areas of confusion and misconceptions that otherwise might lead to erratic or erroneous medication intake.

The patient and his family must realize that the medicine will not take immediate effect. Although some medicines do become fully effective within one to two weeks, many take as long as two to three weeks to manifest their full effect. The patient, the family, and the physician must learn to wait out this full time in order to allow the drug a chance to work; many effective drugs have been discarded prematurely because of impatience. Also, changing drugs every few days not only lessens the chances for good seizure control, but also increases the chances for drug reactions, and may even aggravate the seizure problem, as well as the functioning difficulties. The patient and family also must be aware that during the first two weeks or so of the new medicine the patient may be overly sensitive to it. He may seem less alert, sleepy, irritable, excitable, or overly active. Usually these problems fade away as the body adjusts to the new drug. Sometimes they can be avoided by beginning with a small dose and gradually building up to the average dose over a two- to three-week period; however, a gradual build-up tends to delay the full protection usually gained by a week or two. Finally, if the patient and family are warned honestly about the possibility of side effects, some of which may occur before the follow-up visit, they can contact the physician when an allergic reaction does appear, before it becomes bad. For example, phenobarbital not infrequently causes a little measle-like rash, but it is not serious. However, the drug rashes from many other drugs are more worrisome. If the physician has the confidence of the patient and has been honest and informative about the new medicine, he will be notified about these rashes or other drug reactions as early as possible.

ADJUSTING THE MEDICINE

There are three critical times when the patient should be re-checked by the physician:

1. About three weeks after a new drug has been begun or a major change has been made in the medications, and thereafter.
2. At least once or twice a year, for monitoring the quality of general functioning, seizure control, and any possible drug reactions or emerging problems related to the epilepsy.
3. Whenever there is any concern regarding a possible adverse drug reaction or a change in the seizure pattern.

Patients with focal seizures, those taking more risky drugs, or those with other problems also need to be followed more closely.

The Three-Week Check-up and Later Check-ups

Generally, a new drug or a change in the dosage of an ongoing medication will have achieved its full effect by the end of three weeks. The patient should have recovered from the initial two weeks of sensitivity to a new medicine. Any drug reactions may be beginning to emerge around the second week, although drug rashes tend to appear slightly earlier. The re-examination consists of a review of the effects of the anticonvulsant on the seizures, alertness, behavior, learning, and coordination, as well as a screen for any rashes or other side effects. The examination checks for any side reactions, such as unsteadiness, slurred speech, drowsiness, rashes, yellow jaundice, bruising or bleeding tendencies, enlargement of any body organs, or puffiness of the hands, feet, or face.

Laboratory

The laboratory screen varies depending on the type of drug selected (see Table 9.2). The main laboratory tests consist of a complete blood count (in-

Table 9.2. Basic laboratory evaluations[a]

	Laboratory Test			
Drug	Blood Count (CBC plus)	Urinalysis	Kidney Tests	Liver Function
Barbiturate	12 mo.			(12 mo.)
Dilantin	12 mo.	12 mo.		12 mo.
Tegretol[b]	3 mo.	3 mo.	3 mo.	3 mo.
Minor Meds	6 mo.[c]	6 mo.[c]	6 mo.	6 mo.

[a] At 3 to 4 weeks after beginning a drug and thereafter.

[b] With new drugs, such as Tegretol, Clonipin, and perhaps Valproate, more frequent checks may be needed.

[c] With Tridione and perhaps Zarontin, the blood and urine should be checked monthly for the first year.

Table 9.3. Laboratory concerns and indications of findings

Study	Watch and Repeat	Stop Medication
White Blood Cell Count (WBC)	Below 4,000	Below 2,500–3,000
PMN Count (% × WBC count)	Below 3,000	Below 2,500
Red Blood Cell Count		
Hematocrit (Hct.)	Less than 32%	Less than 30%
Hemoglobin (Hgb.)	Less than 11 g	Less than 10 g
Reticulocyte count (Retic.)	Less than 0.3%	Less than 0.1%
Platelet Count (Plt.)	Less than 100,000	Less than 70,000
Protein in Urine	+	+ + or greater

cluding platelets and reticulocytes) and an examination of the urine. Usually, tests for kidney function and liver function are performed annually or more often depending on the drugs being taken. Periodic checking of these chemistries should be performed in difficult-to-control seizure patients, patients on more than one or two drugs, patients with a history of liver or kidney problems, or patients on drugs that have the potential to produce such problems.

The initial testing is performed at the three-week visit made in followup to the medicine change; thereafter, re-checks are done on an annual basis. With new drugs for which we have less experience and fewer data on possible side effects, and with some of the drugs known to be at increased risk for certain problems, the laboratory studies may be advisable more frequently.

When a laboratory test comes back abnormal and if there is no other apparent reason for the disturbance, such as an infection, bleeding, or some unrelated problem, the laboratory test may need to be repeated. If the laboratory test is sufficiently abnormal to be of a great concern (see Table 9.3), the drug should be stopped.

Anticonvulsant Levels

Monitoring the serum levels of the anticonvulsant drugs has become an important part of the treatment of epilepsy. Monitoring should be performed at least two or three times during the initial phases of adjustment to the medicine; spot-checks should be made periodically thereafter and certainly whenever there is any concern that the level may be too high or too low. There are several systems of measurement presently popular, including the gas liquid chromatography (GLC) method and EMIT System, which is an immunoassay system that can be run quickly on small quantities of blood. At present these tests cover a wide range of reliability and cost, with some labs charging up to or more than five times the reasonable costs and some results being greater than 200% in error. A strong effort is being made to overcome these errors and cost discrepancies.

The blood levels indicate whether the drug content is within the range expected to control seizures. If it is too low, it suggests that the patient is not taking or is not absorbing the medication or that he is metabolizing it more rapidly than anticipated. If the level is too high, it suggests or confirms that the patient is at risk for intoxication side reactions and seizure recurrence.

In addition to several spot-checks, there are certain times when tests of anticonvulsant blood levels should be ordered. These are: 1) to see if the patient is taking the prescribed medicine; 2) to establish an adequate blood level when the actual levels do not agree with the calculated expectation, as with Dilantin in young children and infants; 3) to adjust medications when signs of toxicity appear despite relatively low doses; 4) to determine the offending drug when two or more anticonvulsants are prescribed simultaneously and side effects or toxicity appears; 5) to be sure that the prescribed dose is adequate when seizures continue despite seemingly high drug doses; 6) to differentiate between symptoms related to an overly strong dose of medicine and those due to other causes; 7) to balance the drug levels throughout the day, particularly when only one or two doses per day are under consideration; and 8) to check for possible intoxication in young children or handicapped individuals in whom early signs of toxicity may not be apparent.

Drug levels are not the final arbitrator; they serve only as guidelines. Some patients maintain seizure control despite anticonvulsant blood levels below the desired minimum. Some patients seem to tolerate a medicine without apparent side effects despite a blood level above the maximum dosage usually tolerated; however, these patients should be watched carefully. If the drug is effective without any side effects, it may be best to continue that dosage despite the blood level reports.

SPECIAL SITUATIONS

Stomach Upsets

When a child is vomiting, he may not be able to keep down his medicines. Skipping a meal or two and then beginning small amounts of clear liquids may help settle his stomach. This mild diet should be continued for a day or so. The anticonvulsants may need to be delayed for several doses until the child can retain liquids; then they can be tried with a few extra doses to make up for the missed medications. If more severe vomiting occurs, the physician may be able to give a medication to control the vomiting; he can also give a shot of the anticonvulsant in place of the oral dose. More severe or longer vomiting may require hospitalization for intravenous fluids and injections of the anticonvulsant.

Missed Medication

No matter whether it is due to forgetfulness, carelessness, or vomiting, the missing of medication can be catastrophic. It is one of the commoner causes of prolonged seizures. Missing a dose of a faster-acting drug, such as Celontin, or missing the single daily dosage of any of the slower-acting drugs, such as phenobarbital or Dilantin, can result in a significant dip in the blood levels. If there is any concern that a dose has been forgotten, it is usually safe to give another dose. Even if it turns out to be an extra dose, it will do no more than make the patient slightly sleepy or unsteady for a brief period of time.

Hospitalization for Surgery

When a patient is hospitalized for a major diagnostic procedure or for surgery, there frequently is a period, lasting from hours to a few days, during which the patient is allowed nothing by mouth (NPO). During this time many of the anticonvulsants can be given by shots beneath the skin, into the muscle, or into the veins, or by intravenous fluids. For medications that cannot be administered by shots or intravenously, an extra dose or two can be given during the night prior to the NPO period. Then, as soon as the patient is allowed to take fluids again by mouth, he can begin his daily medicines again, with a few extra doses added over the next few days to make up for the omitted drugs and to restore adequate blood levels.

With hospitalization, close attention must be paid in order to continue the patient on the same dose that he was taking at home, unless deliberate adjustments are made. It may be wise to check blood levels when a prolonged hospitalization is being contemplated. Care must be taken to avoid missing doses inadvertently during the surgical periods or in transfers from one service or floor to another. At the time of surgery or any major procedure the anesthetist should have Valium and phenobarbital ready to be given intravenously should the stress of the procedure trigger a seizure.

Expectations

If a properly used drug is going to be effective, one may expect seizure control within three months of the beginning of therapy. If good control has not been obtained by this time, provided the medication was properly prescribed and used, the chances are not high that the medication will ultimately prove effective. The primary reasons for a poor response are: 1) misdiagnosis of the type of seizure, 2) overlooking the cause of the seizure, 3) poor drug selection, 4) inappropriate drug prescribing (including strength, form, and timing), 5) reactions between drugs, 6) poor patient cooperation, 7) changing medication too rapidly or too frequently, or 8) overtreating the patient.

If the seizures continue after an appropriately prescribed drug has been begun, the drug dose can be worked up slowly to the maximally tolerated dose. If this does not result in control, the physician then should lower the dosage to the minimal dose that still is effective. With some drugs this may prove to be no medication at all. Often the physician will begin another drug simultaneously. Changes in medication should not be rushed. A change should not be made any more frequently than ten days to two weeks with severe, frequent seizure problems and with anticonvulsants that have a rapid turnover in the body. In general, it is best to wait at least three weeks between each change.

It is obviously easier to judge the response to medication in patients who have frequent seizures than with those who have infrequent sporadic attacks. Sometimes, having the patient keep track of the seizures on a calender may help to note both the type and the time of the attacks. This may reveal that the pattern is not the same as that reported by the patient.

ADDITION OF A SECOND OR EVEN A THIRD AND FOURTH DRUG

If the first drug produces some degree of improvement at the most effective and most tolerated dose but does not control the seizure completely, it may be time to add a second drug. If the first drug produces signs of intoxication when control is achieved or neared, a second drug may help with control and allow the intoxication to be avoided. If the second drug is from a different chemical family than the first, the good effects of the two may be complementary, whereas the potential bad effects are not additive. For example, with focal or generalized motor seizure problems, one may choose to add Dilantin to the phenobarbital or Mysoline already in use, whereas with a typical absence attack Zarontin may be the ideal second drug. With atypical absence, akinetic, or myoclonic seizures, Clonipin may be the added drug. The patient and family are concerned that the two drugs will be too strong together. Reassuring them that one drug acts in one way and the other drug acts in a different way will help overcome this concern. In beginning the second drug, one adjusts the first drug to the best dosage and then begins the second drug, following the same approaches as used with the beginning of the first drug.

Anticonvulsants have some cross-reactivity with other drugs and with other anticonvulsants (see Table 9.4). Sometimes the drug levels end up higher than expected and sometimes lower. The results may vary with some combinations. When multiple drugs are used together, blood measurements can be most useful. Obviously, when drugs of the same or similar families are used together, there tends to be cumulative effect. Since both phenobarbital and Mysoline result in phenobarbital in the bloodstream, using both together may result in an elevated barbiturate blood level (see Table 9.5).

Table 9.4. Anticonvulsant choices

First Drug

SEIZURE TYPE:	GENERALIZED MOTOR FOCAL PSYCHOMOTOR	ATYPICAL ABSENCE AKINETIC MYOCLONIC	TYPICAL ABSENCE
Second Drug	Dilantin	Clonipin or Valium Valproate Celontin or Zarontin	Zarontin Tridione Clonipin Valproate Celontin
Third Drug	Tegretol	Diamox	Diamox
Alternatives	Celontin Valproate	Dilantin Ketogenic Diet	Ketogenic Diet

A barbiturate → Mysoline

Table 9.5. Interactions of anticonvulsants: Effects on blood levels

Blood Level of Drug	Influencing Drug							
	Barbiturates & Mysoline	Dilantin	Tegretol	Celontin & Zarontin	Tridione	Clonipin & Valium	Valproate	Diamox
Barbiturates and Mysoline	+		+			+	+	
Dilantin	±	+	−			+	−	
Tegretol		+	+	+				
Zarontin and Celontin		±	±	+				
Tridione					+			
Clonipin and Valium						+		
Valproate						+	+	
Diamox								+

Some combinations are especially useful. A barbiturate and Zarontin or another "minor medication" together often control absence seizures and protect against a major seizure. Sometimes the combination of lower doses of Zarontin and Tridione, two minor medications, will be more effective than either drug alone. Celontin seems especially helpful when there is a mixed seizure disorder, such as atypical absence and temporal lobe attacks or multifocal seizures. The combination of Mysoline, Dilantin, and Clonipin may be effective with myoclonic attacks.

If satisfactory control of the seizures is achieved with the combination, continue both medications. If the control is not satisfactory despite adjustments, a third and rarely even a fourth or fifth anticonvulsant can be added, following the same procedures and precautions as with the other drugs. However, multiple drugs are usually not necessary and tend to be overused.

Often a simpler drug combination of fewer medications can be more effective and less toxic. Piling drugs on one after another often represents only a desperate effort to control the attacks. Such measures may only be needed with severe, uncontrolled mixed seizure problems and then only if simpler approaches prove ineffective. In general, if a seizure problem cannot be controlled with appropriate medication within six months, there is little chance that total control will ever be achieved.

SUBSTITUTION OF ONE DRUG FOR ANOTHER

If a seizure does not respond to a drug or if the patient cannot tolerate a drug, begin another medication and then gradually discontinue the offending agent while the new medicine is building up. Do this slowly and cautiously, taking at least two to three weeks to allow the protective effects of the new drug to build up before making further changes. If one drug does not work, gradually switch to another. Successful control may depend on the persistence of the physician in searching for the right drug or drug combination. Switching too rapidly or too soon is to be avoided, for it is more apt to be harmful than helpful.

WITHDRAWAL: GRADUALLY DISCONTINUING A DRUG

There are four situations in which a drug is discontinued: 1) acutely in a severe drug reaction, 2) any time a drug is felt to be ineffective, 3) if the patient is reluctant to take the medicine, or 4) after three or four years or more of complete seizure control.

Acute Withdrawal for a Toxic Reaction

If the patient experiences a severe allergic reaction to a drug, such as a bad rash, very low blood count, or liver or kidney problems, the drug must be stopped. There is a high risk of a seizure breakthrough during the period following the abrupt withdrawal. The patient often is hospitalized both for treatment of the reaction and for precautionary observation for a breakthrough seizure. The offending drug should never be used again. Drugs of a similar chemical structure may also tend to cause a similar reaction and must be tried very cautiously if at all. Since all anticonvulsants have similar chemical structures, any replacement anticonvulsant may potentially trigger the reaction, especially during the acute allergic period. It would be most desirable to wait two or even three months before beginning a new drug, to allow the allergic reactivity to settle down. Often this is not possible. If a new anticonvulsant is needed, it is best to select one that is chemically dissimilar from the offending agent and one that has a low risk for allergic reactions. The drug should be begun cautiously and monitored closely. If a reaction does occur, yet is mild and caught early, sometimes it may be continued by using antihistamines and even steroids during the reactive period to suppress the allergy until the body is able to tolerate the new drug.

Ineffective Medicines

If a medicine is felt to have no effect or to have lost its previously good effect, as for example Diamox and Valium may tend to do, or if the seizures continue to occur despite the use of multiple medications, it may be valuable to see if the drug is still effective. The goal is to find the smallest dose that is necessary. Slowly begin to withdraw the drugs, one at a time, starting with the most recent drug tried. If the reduction and even discontinuation of the medicine do not result in worsening of the seizure problem, the drug probably was not needed. Sometimes the lowering of a drug dosage or discontinuation results in better seizure control. This may be seen especially with Celontin in cases of "minor seizures." If, however, the drug is still needed at some point following a withdrawal step, the seizures will begin to become worse. If this happens, return the drug to the most effective and best-tolerated dose.

Poor Cooperation in Drug Intake

If the side effects of the drug are more bothersome to the patient than the seizures, if the patient feels that taking the medication is too bothersome or too dangerous, or if the patient is emotionally unstable and cannot be trusted to take his medication, it may be wiser to discontinue the medicine slowly before the patient decides to stop it himself. The danger of severe or prolonged seizures from erratic drug intake or the abrupt stoppage of medicines is far greater than the recurrence of seizures following a controlled discontinuation of the medicine. It may be best to wait until the patient and his family are better able to cooperate.

Prolonged Seizure Control

When a patient's seizures have been completely controlled for at least three to four years, it may be time to consider discontinuing the medication. (One reason that the physician should be immediately notified of a breakthrough in seizure control is that the breakthrough seizure becomes the new beginning of the three-year control period. If the physician is not told until the next office visit, it only prolongs the treatment.) Since there are realistic risks for recurrence of the seizure, the patient and his family may hesitate to take the chance. A seizure recurrence may be a social catastrophe, especially to the adolescent; it may interfere with school, job, or driving opportunities. The withdrawal should be done at a time convenient to the patient.

Withdrawal must be performed very cautiously, if at all, if there are factors that increase the risk for recurrence. These risk factors include: entry into early puberty, the first seizures occurring after 9 to 10 years of age, a prolonged period (six months or more) of appropriate therapeutic efforts before control over the attacks is gained, focal seizures, seizures caused by a structural defect in the brain, or a mixed seizure disorder. The chances for seizure recurrence are greater in the adult than in the child. Focal or mixed seizure problems are more apt to recur than are generalized motor or especially absence attacks. Patients with a neurologic abnormality on examination are more apt to experience a seizure recurrence than those with a normal neurologic examination. Although a normal EEG is reassuring, the EEG is not helpful in deciding which patients may safely be weaned from their medications and which are at risk for recurrence. An EEG abnormality may persist the remainder of the patient's life without any recurrence of seizures. The best outlook is when the seizure began between ages 4 to 8 years in an otherwise normal child, recurring seldom if ever, and easily controlled by one or two medications.

If a medicine is stopped abruptly, the breakthrough attack is more apt to occur within three to seven days or more after the last dose. If the medicine is discontinued slowly, the greatest risk for recurrence is within the first few months and the risk continues for up to two years. After two years, the risk for recurrence is minimal. Sometimes the seizure recurs during the tapering period, indicating that the medication is still needed.

Approach Drugs must be withdrawn very slowly and cautiously, one drug at a time, beginning with the most risky drug, in order to avoid seizure recurrence or irritability, agitation, or hyperexcitability due to the changing medications. With milder seizure problems (those seizures easily controlled with average doses of common anticonvulsants) the tapering can be done over a one- to two-year period. With simple absence attacks the withdrawal period may be even shorter, over a six- to twelve-month period.

With more severe seizure problems, it may be wiser to reduce the medications gradually over a period of three to four years. Major seizure medications, such as the barbiturates, Dilantin, and Tegretol, may be tapered over a one- to two-year period each, whereas the minor seizure medications may be withdrawn more rapidly, over a six- to twelve-month period each. The order of withdrawal of the medications should be the reverse of the order of adding the medications, in order to discontinue the more risky drugs before the safest. Usually the last drug to be discontinued is the barbiturate.

Recurrence If a seizure recurs during or after the withdrawal period, therapy should be begun again at the previously effective drug dose. Unless there is a good reason for the breakthrough, the next attempt at discontinuation, if ever, should be done only after an appropriate period of control and should be done very slowly and very cautiously! Any further recurrence suggests a dependence on the medication for seizure control, meaning that the patient probably should remain on the medication for an extended period, most likely the rest of his life.

CONCLUSION

Seizure control is centered on a one-drug-at-a-time approach, based on careful drug selection, taking into account the seizure type and the effectiveness and toxicity of each drug, practicing a gradual build-up and close monitoring of the seizure control and patient's functioning, and ending in a slow and cautious discontinuation of anticonvulsant medication. Patience and careful monitoring are necessary. Seizure control should never be obtained at the cost of optimal daily functioning. Seizure control should never be thought of as the addition of medications when seizures occur; it is best done by helping the patient function at his best level, with drugs being one of many tools to help achieve this goal.

REFERENCES AND SUGGESTED READINGS

Aird, R. B., and D. M. Woodbury. 1974. The Management of Epilepsy. Charles C Thomas, Springfield, Illinois. 448 pp.

Berman, P. B. 1976. Management of seizure disorders with anticonvulsant drugs: Current concepts. Pediatr. Clin. North Am. 23:443-459.

Brett, E. 1977. Implications of measuring anticonvulsant blood levels in epilepsy. Dev. Med. Child Neurol. 19:245-251.

Bruya, M. A., and R. H. Bolin. 1976. Epilepsy: A controllable disease. Classification and diagnosis of seizures. Am. J. Nurs. 76:388-397.

Castle, G. F., and L. S. Fishman. 1973. Seizures. Pediatr. Clin. North Am. 20: 819-835.

(The) Commission for the Control of Epilepsy and Its Consequences. 1977. Plan for Nationwide Action on Epilepsy. DHEW Publication No. (NIH) 78-276. Office of Scientific and Health Reports, NINCDS-NIH Bethesda, Maryland. 4 volumes.

Holowach, J., D. L. Thurston, and J. O'Leary. 1972. Prognosis in childhood epilepsy: Follow-up of 148 cases in which therapy had been suspended after prolonged anticonvulsant control. New Engl. J. Med. 286:169-174.

Kutt, H. 1975. Interactions of antiepileptic drugs. Epilepsia 16:393-402.

Livingston, S. 1972. Comprehensive Management of Epilepsy in Infancy, Childhood and Adolescence. Charles C Thomas, Springfield, Illinois. 657 pp.

Livingston, S. 1973. Seizure disorders. In: S. S. Gellis and B. Kagan (eds.), Current Pediatric Therapy, Ed. 6, pp. 78-92. W. B. Saunders Company, Philadelphia.

Menkes, J. H. 1976. Diagnosis and treatment of minor motor seizures. Pediatr. Clin. North Am. 23:435-442.

Painter, M. J., C. Pippenger, H. MacDonald, and W. Pitlick. 1978. Phenobarbital and Dilantin levels in neonates with seizures. J. Pediatr. 92:315-319.

Richens, A. 1976. Drug Treatment of Epilepsy. Year Book Medical Publishers, Inc., Chicago. 176 pp.

Sands, H., and F. C. Minters. 1977. The Epilepsy Fact Book. F. A. Davis Co., Philadelphia. 116 pp.

Sholl, M. L. 1966. Epilepsy in Children. In: H. F. Conn (ed.), Current Therapy, pp. 574-581. W. B. Saunders Company, Philadelphia.

Singer, H. S., and J. M. Freeman. 1975. Seizures in adolescents. Med. Clin. North Am. 59:1461-1472.

Solomon, G. E., and F. Plum. 1976. Clinical Management of Seizures. W. B. Saunders Company, Philadelphia. 152 pp.

10
ANTICONVULSANT SIDE EFFECTS

No drug is completely safe. The physician, the patient, and his family should all be aware of the potential side effects of a medicine. If the side effects are detected early enough, more serious problems may be avoided. Subtle side effects may be overlooked, and yet these reactions may become more handicapping than the seizures.

Most side effects are reversible and not dangerous. Unsteadiness, slight incoordination, drowsiness, overgrowth of the gums and hair, mild rashes, slurred speech, or visual complaints, although bothersome, are not dangerous. Many of these can be avoided. Infrequent but dangerous side effects include those affecting the blood, the skin, the liver, or the kidneys. If neglected and allowed to progress, these may become fatal.

There are four major types of drug reactions. An *intoxication* is a reversible condition due to taking too strong a dose of medication. An *allergy* is a physiological reaction to a drug the body cannot tolerate. An *idiosyncrasy* is an unexpected, bothersome drug effect that seldom is dangerous. A *malformation* occurs when a drug taken during pregnancy has an effect on the unborn child.

INTOXICATION

The drug-intoxicated individual is taking more medicine than his system can handle. The dose prescribed may be too strong. The patient may be taking too much of the medicine on his own. He may be extra-efficient in absorbing the medicine into his body. His system may be slow at removing the drug from the body.

Levels of Intoxication

There is a desired concentration for each anticonvulsant in the bloodstream. Within this range, most patients can take the drug without side effects. If the levels fall below this range, the seizures may break through. If the levels rise above this range, most patients begin to experience side effects, depending on how high above the maximum level the drug rises. Some individuals can tolerate more than the expected amount of a drug in their blood without side effects; some individuals experience side effects even in the usual "safe" range. Thus the final decision is based both on the clinical observation and on the blood levels.

In the upper half of the effective yet tolerated blood level range and higher, the eyes may exhibit brief jerky movements (nystagmus). This sign suggests that the patient's blood level is at least in the adequate range, if not too high.

Most anticonvulsants follow the same pattern of intoxication symptoms, although there are two different onsets. With most anticonvulsants, in the first stage of a mild intoxication the patient is not as alert as he normally is. His thinking and performance are slowed. His work or his school performance may deteriorate. With Dilantin, however, the initial sign of intoxication is that of drunkenness rather than drowsiness. The Dilantin-drunk patient cannot walk a straight line without staggering unsteadily. His speech may be slurred. With either form of mild intoxication the patient may be more apt to experience seizures again.

In moderate intoxication the patient becomes both drowsy and drunk. He is clumsy. Abnormal movements, such as tremors, jerks, twisting, or abnormal posturing may be seen. The gaze may no longer be focused. The patient tends to fall asleep easily. The blood level of the anticonvulsant may be as high as twice the normal level.

The severely intoxicated patient staggers and lurches around in a half-asleep stupor. He falls easily. He cannot focus his eyes. He may be nauseated and vomit easily. His blood pressure may be low. He breathes slowly and shallowly.

The profoundly intoxicated patient is in a deep sleep or coma. His blood pressure is dangerously low; his breathing is very slow and shallow if indeed he is breathing. He may need to be on an artificial respirator to keep him alive until his blood level drops. His brainwave test may be nearly flat. Indeed, he may seem dead, but within 24 hours both he and his EEG will begin to show signs of recovery, provided that intensive support has been maintained.

Initial Intoxication

In the first 10 or 12 days after beginning a new drug, the patient may seem irritable, agitated, emotionally labile, or intoxicated. He may be hyperactive. These signs often clear within three weeks, when the body has adjusted to more efficient handling of the medication and becomes less sensitive to it. This reaction is especially true with Mysoline, Clonipin, and Tegretol, but it may be seen with all anticonvulsants. Initial sensitivity may be avoided by beginning with a smaller dosage and gradually building up to the desired dosage as the patient tolerates the medicine. However, if the reaction is too extreme or persists beyond the second or third week, the patient may be overly sensitive and not able to take the medication. The drug may need to be continued at a much lower dosage. The drug will probably have to be discontinued.

Acute Overdosage

A confused or depressed patient or a young child may accidently or purposefully swallow a large amount of anticonvulsants at once. If this fact is discovered within an hour or so, the stomach may be pumped out or vomiting may be induced, so that part of the overdosage may be retrieved before it is absorbed. Often the patient must be admitted to the hospital for support and further investigation. It is important to find out the circumstances behind the taking of the drugs, so that a recurrence may be prevented. A blood level is not as important as the identification of the drug(s) by a screen of the blood, the urine, and the stomach contents.

Sometimes after a severe intoxication or a massive dose of an anticonvulsant, the neurologic symptoms may improve but they may not completely clear. Unsteadiness may persist after an overly large dose of Dilantin.

Chronic Intoxication

Prolonged use of anticonvulsant drugs at levels above the usual range can lead to a deterioration of intelligence, behavior, or emotional stability. The high blood levels may depress the making of blood in the bone marrow. The patient may seem retarded, uncoordinated, and unsteady; a degenerative disease of the nervous system may be suspected. Rather than improving, the seizures may be worsened. During pregnancy, the unborn child may be at increased risk for a malformation.

The signs and symptoms of chronic intoxication may be delayed, subtle, and overlooked. Consequently it is wise to measure anticonvulsant blood levels not only when beginning the drug, but also periodically thereafter, as a double-check against a chronic intoxication even when major drug changes have not been made. The functioning of the patient in school or at work also should be watched for any deterioration that might suggest a drug reaction.

The infant and young child are both erratic in absorption and widely variable in the metabolism of some of the anticonvulsant drugs. Dilantin may be poorly absorbed in the very young child; the resultant blood levels may vary widely from child to child. Dilantin blood levels must be followed closely in the infant and preschool child.

Some people clear drugs from their systems rapidly, whereas others may be exceptionally slow at clearing the medicine. Consequently, an average dose may result in a very low or a very high blood level, depending on the clearance rate. A slow or a fast clearance rate may be a familial trait, and it may affect other drugs besides those for epilepsy treatment. The anticonvulsant must be adjusted to the desired blood level range and to the patient's best functional state.

Drug Interactions

When two or more drugs are given together, one drug may speed up or slow down the turnover of the other drug in the body. This interaction between drugs, be they two anticonvulsants or an anticonvulsant and another drug, is fairly common. It may not always be detrimental. The interactions may vary between people. The most common anticonvulsant drug involved in drug interactions is Dilantin.

When a new drug is added and the patient is already on another drug, changes in the seizure pattern and the appearance of side effects may be due to alterations produced by either drug. For example, adding phenobarbital to Dilantin may cause the Dilantin level to drop or occasionally to rise. Stopping the phenobarbital and keeping on Dilantin alone is more apt to cause a rise in the blood Dilantin level than a drop. Consequently, before either drug is labeled as the cause of the symptoms, or before either drug can be credited for the improvement or worsening of the seizures, blood levels for both drugs must be checked.

Management of Intoxication

If the intoxication is mild or moderate, the drug dose needs to be lowered. It is usually wise to obtain an initial drug level measurement to be sure that the drug level is too high. If the intoxication is moderately severe or higher, the drug needs to be discontinued until the level drops to a milder range of intoxication. Rather than aggravating the seizure tendency by suddenly stopping medication, discontinuing the medication will improve control, unless it is stopped for too lengthy a period. It is probably wise to restart the medication when the intoxication symptoms still are mildly present, so that the drug levels will not drop below the therapeutic range. The severely intoxicated patient will have to be hospitalized for intensive support and therapy.

Seizures versus Intoxication

When a patient appears drowsy and unsteady and exhibits slurred speech, the cause may be drug intoxication or the breakthrough of minor or missed seizures. The seizures could be due to overmedication or undermedication. Checking the blood anticonvulsant levels and carefully watching the patient for small seizures will help determine whether the medications need to be increased or decreased.

Undermedication

The blood anticonvulsant levels may be too low to protect against a seizure. This may be because the dose prescribed or given is too small, inaccurately measured, or given in a poorly absorbable and mixable liquid form. Rarely, an error in filling the prescription may be made, but the patient familiar with his medication should note this. The patient may not want his seizures controlled because it would mean the loss of extra attention, benefits, or leisure, implying obligation to work. He may forget his medicines because he has problems accepting his epilepsy.

People vary in their absorption of medicine and also in how they metabolize medication within their body. Slowed absorption and rapid metabolism may lead to low blood levels. Giving other drugs simultaneously or taking the drugs with meals may affect the absorption.

In the hospital, the route of administration of the drug is important. A quicker and higher dosage can be obtained by giving the medication intravenously than by giving it as an injection into the muscle or beneath the skin. The latter injection, providing it is a medication that does not crystallize out or produce inflammation, will reach a less dangerous level but last for 4 to 6 hours. When the patient is inactive and has poor circulation or cold limbs the absorption may be delayed. Giving medicine as a rectal suppository is undesirable because the absorption is erratic.

Although frequently low blood levels are caused by not taking the medication, the patient is not always to blame. When a breakthrough seizure occurs, monitoring the blood levels with samples drawn before giving booster injections may indicate the cause. The cure for the problem may be to alter the dosage prescribed, to change the form of the medicine, to change procedures for giving the medication, and to counsel the patient and his family about why the drug is necessary.

ALLERGIES

An allergic reaction to a drug means that the patient cannot tolerate the drug at any dosage. The reaction can be dangerous and even fatal. Many drug reactions labeled drug allergies are not true allergies, they are intoxications or idiosyncratic reactions. Allergies, unlike the other types of drug reactions, are not related to the strength of the medication, since as little as one dose may trigger the reaction. In an allergy, the offending drug combines with a body protein; it is the combination that triggers the body response, i.e., an allergic reaction. It usually takes from one to two weeks for a reaction to occur, although if the patient has had previous exposures to the medication, the reaction may occur within minutes.

There are three types of allergic reactions, the acute anaphylactic reaction, a serum sickness hypersensitivity reaction, and a delayed organ system reaction.

Acute Anaphylactic Reaction

If a patient has been exposed to a drug or a similar medication previously, an anaphylactic reaction may appear within minutes to hours after the patient receives the medication as an injection or within hours to a few days after he begins to take the medication by mouth. Often, the quicker the onset is, the more severe the reaction is. The patient may feel agitated, irritable, jittery, or anxious. He may appear pale or flushed, and often he breaks out in red blotches and hives. His face may swell. He may have problems breathing, as if he were having an asthmatic attack or croup. His heart rate may be fast but his blood pressure often may drop to dangerously low levels. He may be confused and drowsy, or he may lose consciousness. When this happens, he often needs intensive support, including oxygen, medications, and proper positioning to bring his blood pressure up, epinephrine to overcome his breathing spasms, and antihistamines or steroids to slow the reaction.

Serum Sickness Hypersensitivity Reactions

A serum sickness reaction is more apt to begin about two to three weeks or more after a medicine is begun; it may begin earlier if the patient has been on the drug previously. There are three types of reactions, a basic hypersensitivity reaction sometimes called a drug fever, a more complex form sometimes called a pseudo-lymphoma syndrome, and a still more complex form sometimes called a pseudo-rheumatoid or pseudo-collagen disorder syndrome, because they mimic these diseases. These hypersensitivity syndromes are outlined in Table 10.1.

Basic Hypersensitivity Reaction Any anticonvulsant may trigger a basic hypersensitivity reaction, consisting of a fever (drug fever) of unexplained origin, often accompanied by drowsiness or confusion, mildly enlarged lymph glands, and a skin rash. There may be accompanying allergic reactions of the blood, the liver, or the kidney.

Pseudo-Lymphoma Syndrome Most of the anticonvulsants, except for the simple barbiturates, may cause a syndrome that not only contains the primary features of a basic hypersensitivity reaction, but also is noted for significant enlargement of the lymph nodes, the liver, and the spleen. The joints frequently ache. Initially, concern is that the patient has infectious mononucleosis or a tumor of the lymph nodes, until a full investigation reveals the true cause.

Table 10.1. Hypersensitivity syndromes

	Simple	Pseudo-Lymphoma	Pseudo-rheumatoid
Barbiturates and	+	0	0
Mysoline	+ +	+ + +	+ +
Dilantin	+ + +	+ + +	+ + +
Tegretol	+ +	?	?
Zarontin and Celontin	+ +	+ +	+ + +
Tridione	+ +	+ + +	+ +
Clonipin and Valium	+ +	?	?
Valproate	+ +	?	?
Diamox	+ +	?	?

Pseudo-Rheumatoid or Pseudo-Collagen Disorder Syndrome The pseudo-rheumatoid syndrome presents with all the features found in the simple hypersensitivity reaction and the pseudo-lymphoma syndrome plus multiple enlarged, tender, warm, and painful joints, a variety of skin rashes, including a butterfly-shaped rash across the cheeks and bridge of the nose, and often inflammation of the blood vessels throughout the body, including the kidney; it is often mistaken for a rheumatoid disorder affecting the collagen connective system, joints, and blood vessels of the body, as seen with systemic lupus erythematosus, polyarteritis nodosa, or rheumatoid arthritis. The drug seems to trigger the body to react with unleashed immunity against its own tissue. Stopping the medication may cause these three syndromes to subside.

Delayed Systemic Reactions

A delayed systemic reaction may occur at any time, but its onset is most usual about a week or two after beginning a new medication. The allergic reaction may involve the skin, the blood, the liver, or the kidneys. This reaction may be limited to any one of these systems, or it may be part of a hypersensitivity reaction, as with serum sickness. Early reactions may be detected at the three-week check-up after beginning the new medication. The specific allergic reactions are listed in Table 10.2.

Table 10.2. Specific allergic reactions

	Skin Rash	Blood	Liver	Kidney
Barbiturate and Mysoline	+	±	?	0
Dilantin	+ + +	+ + +	+ + +	+
Tegretol	+ +	+ + +	+ +	+ +
Zarontin and Celontin	+ +	+ + +	+	+ + +
Tridione	+ +	+ + +	+ +	+ + +
Valium and Clonipin	+	+	+	±
Valproate	+	?	+	?
Diamox	+	+ +	+	+

Rashes Any drug may cause any type of rash of any degree of severity at any time. Rashes most often begin 10 days or more after beginning a medicine. The rash may be a minor measles-like rash, as is often seen with phenobarbital. With careful monitoring, it may not be necessary to stop the drug or to use an antihistamine unless the rash gets worse. Often it will go away without treatment. A more severe rash, i.e., red blotches and hives, usually is treated with an antihistamine. The drug may need to be stopped. Severe reactions, such as exfoliative dermatitis, when the skin peels and flakes off, or bullous-blistering reactions, especially when they involve the mucous membranes of the eyelids, nose, mouth, and urinary and genital tracts, are dangerous. The drug must be stopped and the reaction must be treated intensively.

The skin may offer clues to other types of reactions. Bruising and bleeding, yellow jaundice, or swelling of the face, hands, and feet may be seen with blood, liver, or kidney problems.

Blood Reactions A drug allergy may affect the white blood cells (WBC), which fight off infections, the red blood cells (RBC), which carry oxygen, or the platelets, which promote blood clotting. The reaction may prevent production of all of these elements in the bone marrow, as is most often seen with a toxic accumulation of a drug. An allergic reaction may affect the cells as they circulate in the bloodstream, usually causing one type of cell to stick together, break up, and be destroyed.

A leukopenia or neutropenia, or the more severe form, an agranulocytosis, indicates that the white blood cells are either being destroyed or not made. The patient is more prone to infection. He may develop mouth ulcers.

An anemia indicates a lack of red blood cells due to underproduction, an excessive loss due to bleeding, or an early destruction and removal of the circulating RBC. If the problem is a lack of production, the number of immature RBC, the reticulocytes, may be decreased; in blood loss due to destruction or hemorrhage, the retics are usually high, since the body is trying to replace the lost red blood cells. The patient often feels fatigued and looks pale.

Thrombocytopenia means a lack of platelets. The patient is apt to experience easy bruising and excessive bleeding. A viral infection can cause a thrombocytopenia, an anemia, or a drop in the white blood cell count that may be mistaken for a drug reaction.

A pancytopenia, or lack of all of the blood types, more often is due to an underproduction in the bone marrow; it may occasionally be due to a severe allergic reaction. All the symptoms of the separate blood type deficiencies occur, only they may occur in steps, since some blood cell types live longer than others. In succession the patient may experience bruising, infections, mouth ulcers, pallor, fatigue, and then severe bleeding. These symptoms may appear as early as seven days after a new drug is begun, although the onset is usually later and the course rather long.

Drug Hepatitis An allergic reaction of the liver may affect either the liver cells, disrupting liver function, or the tubules draining the bile from the liver. Disturbed liver functions show up as elevated liver enzymes and bleeding problems due to depressed blood clotting factors. There is often a tendency for a transient rise in liver enzymes whenever a new drug is begun. Clinically the patient may have a large tender liver and his skin and eyes may appear yellow (jaundiced).

Kidney Problems An allergic nephrosis or nephrotic syndrome results in leaky kidney tubules. Protein leaks out excessively into the urine, leaving a deficiency of protein in the blood. This results in puffy swelling (edema) of the hands, face, or feet. Another reaction involves the blood vessels of the kidney as a hemorrhagic nephritis. The urine shows an excess of red blood cells and clusters of red cells and casts of protein. Kidney function is impaired.

Management of Allergic Problems

The patient, the physician, the family, and all persons working with the seizure patient should be aware of the early signs of an allergic reaction. Screening the blood and urine at three weeks, periodically thereafter, or whenever a reaction is suspected may help detect early reactions. If a blood, blood chemistry, or urine test is suspicious but not conclusive, it should be repeated. If the reaction is mild, it may be possible to continue the drug if the reaction can be controlled with Benadryl. If the reaction is more severe, the drug and all similar drugs must be stopped; the reaction itself must be suppressed with antihistamine drugs or steroids until it has run its course. The offending drug should not be used again. Similar drugs should be avoided whenever possible; if they are used, they must be used with caution. It is desirable to wait as long as possible after a drug reaction before beginning a new drug, since the body may be so hypersensitive that it may expand the reaction to include the new drug also. If waiting at least a month or two is not possible, then the new drug should be as chemically different from the offending drug, and as non-allergenic, as possible.

IDIOSYNCRATIC REACTIONS

An idiosyncratic reaction is an unexpected reaction that is bothersome but rarely dangerous. The reaction tends to relate to the strength of the medication but the relationship is not as direct as with an intoxication. The reaction usually appears soon after a medication is begun, or else it may slowly build up over a long period of time. Reactions that begin with the introduction of the drug may persist or may fade away when the body becomes used to the drug, usually within a month or two. The main types of reactions include psychologic disturbances, neurologic symptoms, and other symptoms, such as complaints about the eyes or the stomach.

Psychologic Disturbances

The principal psychologic disturbances include depression or deterioration of learning, intelligence, or behavior, and emotional instability. This can happen with the introduction of the drug or it can be a gradual and chronic effect.

Any drug may produce emotional instability, agitation, irritability, restlessness, excessive crying, temper, or hyperactivity. Phenobarbital especially, but not exclusively, has been associated with these symptoms in the elderly, in the brain-damaged child, and in the normal person. Sometimes milder forms of this behavior are transient and fade after two or three weeks. More severe and persistent hyperactive or emotional behaviors may be accentuations of previous tendencies brought out by the drug or may even be a pre-existing problem that is later blamed on the drug. If phenobarbital is felt to be the culprit, sometimes Gemonil or Mebaral can be substituted with less chance of precipitating the same reactions. Otherwise the barbiturate may have to be changed to another type of anticonvulsant.

Some drugs, such as Mysoline, may result in a confusional or very drowsy state, often accompanied by nausea and vomiting even when only one pill has been taken. To avoid this and to test for the possibility, Mysoline is often begun as a very small initial dose for a few days. Some of the anticonvulsants may precipitate more severe psychiatric disturbances, confused thinking, or psychotic reactions.

Within the normal therapeutic range, the anticonvulsant drugs should have little or no effect on learning. The barbiturates may reduce the ability to concentrate for long periods of intensive study. Dilantin, if used as the only drug, may be associated with delays in reading, particularly with focal seizures in a young boy. Various claims have been made for various drugs to be "less disturbing" or even to "improve learning," but these claims have not been substantiated. Sometimes the drugs to which the wonder drug is compared are used at overly strong doses in order to control the seizures, at the cost of alertness, an approach that is undesirable.

With chronic drug usage, even if it is maintained within a normal range, a subtle, slow deterioration of intelligence, emotions, or behaviors may occur. This is especially apt to occur, although infrequently, with Dilantin. The problem usually but not always can be overcome by switching to another anticonvulsant drug. The patient must be seen at least yearly if not more frequently, and should be questioned about his functioning at work or at school, and his emotions and behaviors, in order to avoid this tendency.

Neurologic Reactions

Some patients will present with symptoms of intoxication even though their drug levels are in a normal to low anticonvulsant blood level range. This is an idiosyncratic effect. Mysoline may be especially apt to cause this. Abnormal peculiar jerking, twisting, or bizarre posturing movements may be seen with Dilantin and perhaps with Tegretol. Tegretol and Clonipin have been linked to complaints of dizziness and unsteadiness. Other complaints may include headaches, light-headedness, or unsteadiness. When such problems occur, the drug may be reduced to see if it can be tolerated at a lower level and still be effective.

Other Systemic Complaints

The cosmetic effects of Dilantin may be more disturbing to the adolescent girl than the seizures. These changes, which begin at about two to three months after starting on Dilantin and which last as long as the patient is on Dilantin, include a tendency toward coarsening of the facial features, growth of darker hair on the face and body, and overgrowth of the gums, particularly if the dental care is poor or if the child wears braces. A dentist may be a useful member of the team: dental care can be improved and gum overgrowth can be trimmed back as needed.

Patients on Tegretol, Tridione, Zarontin, and Celontin especially may have eye complaints. Things may seem too bright to them, they may not see clearly, or they may have problems seeing at night. They may develop dark circles under their eyes, but these tend to go away after a month or two.

The GI system is often involved in idiosyncratic reactions. The minor seizure medications, particularly Zarontin, Celontin, and Tridione, may cause hiccups for the first month or so. Some anticonvulsants, such as Mysoline, may lead to a loss of appetite and to vomiting. Some drugs, such as Dilantin or Celontin, may be so irritating to the stomach that the patient complains of abdominal aches, nausea, and often vomiting. Taking the drug at meals, although it tends to reduce the absorption, may overcome this reaction and also serves as a good reminder to take the medication. Antacids may overcome the stomach irritation, but they interfere with the absorption of the drug.

RISKS WITH PREGNANCY

The pregnant woman who is on anticonvulsant drugs in an effort to control her epilepsy is at increased risk for problems in her offspring. These problems include: anemia, hemorrhagic problems of the newborn, and the distinct possibility of malformations and mental retardation. The woman should be aware of these risks.

Anemia

The pregnant mother, and consequently her child, is apt to become anemic when on anticonvulsants. Often the anemia is megaloblastic, i.e., the red blood cells are too large. Since the cause of the anemia is often a lack of folic acid, the problem can be overcome by giving enough folic acid to correct the anemia. However, care should be taken to avoid an excess of this vitamin, which may decrease seizure control. The baby should be checked at birth for possible anemia.

Bleeding Problems

When the mother is on anticonvulsant medications, the newborn infant may have bleeding problems, which may be due to low platelet levels or to immature liver function. All newborn infants born of a mother on anticonvulsant medications should have a complete blood count, including a platelet count; they should also receive a shot of vitamin K.

Malformations

Of rising concern and increasing documentation is the realistic risk of mental retardation and various malformations of offspring born to an epileptic woman on anticonvulsant medications. The most incriminated drugs include Dilantin, Tridione, and the barbiturates, as well as related drugs. Animal studies suggest that most of the other anticonvulsant drugs may also have detrimental influences. The most common malformations include cleft lips and palates, heart defects, and kidney malformations.

Newly identified are a "fetal Dilantin syndrome" and a "fetal Tridione syndrome," and perhaps even a "fetal barbiturate syndrome." These syndromes each have a characteristic facial appearance, individual clusters of minor anomalies, mental retardation in the mild to moderate range, and low-set, malformed ears. The Dilantin syndrome is especially noteworthy for the underdevelopment of the nails at birth; these grow out in the first year. The Tridione syndrome characteristically causes V-shaped eyebrows and folded, floppy ears.

The risks for a malformation may be increased if there is a family history for such malformations and if the mother is over 35 years of age, is diabetic, or has a history of previous stillbirths or miscarriages. These risks should be discussed with the patient whenever a pregnancy is anticipated. If the seizures have been controlled for a period of time, it may be possible and advisable to taper off the medication before the pregnancy occurs. It may also be advisable for the woman taking Tridione or Dilantin to avoid pregnancy. If the patient is on a barbiturate, every effort should be made to maintain a low therapeutic blood level, since higher levels may increase the risks for malformations. The risks may be especially high in the first four to six weeks of pregnancy. When a pregnancy occurs, the simplest and safest drugs should be selected, with as few medications as possible being used. The drug levels should be monitored closely throughout the pregnancy. The physician should anticipate potential pregnancies in the woman of childbearing age and he should make every effort in selecting her treatment to avoid any drug clearly linked with malformations when a safer drug is an available alternative. However, uncontrolled scizures during the pregnancy may carry risk to the fetus; careful and cautious use of anticonvulsant medicines may avoid fetal death or more severe damage.

CONCLUSION

The patient, the physician, and those around the patient should be on guard for any emerging side effects. Periodic monitoring of the blood levels, blood count, blood chemistries, and urine, as well as a full examination at least once a year, may catch an early reaction before lasting damage can be done. Intoxications are overcome by lowering the dosage of the drug. Allergies are treated by stopping the drug permanently and suppressing the allergic reactions with antihistamines and steroids. Idiosyncracies are managed by stopping the drug only if the reaction is too bothersome. During a pregnancy it is advisable to use anticonvulsant medication cautiously and carefully, with frequent monitoring of the anticonvulsant blood levels and checking of the newborn for possible anemia, thrombocytopenia, or bleeding tendencies, as well as for any malformations.

REFERENCES AND SUGGESTED READING

General

Aird, R. B., and D. M. Woodbury. 1974. The Management of Epilepsy. Charles C Thomas, Springfield, Ill. 448 pp.
Livingston, S. 1966. Drug Therapy for Epilepsy. Charles C Thomas, Springfield, Ill. 234 pp.
Meinardi, H., and L. M. K. Stoll. 1974. Side effects of antiepileptic drugs. In: O. Magnus and A. M. Lorentz de Haas (eds.), The Epilepsies, chap. 37, pp. 705-738. P. J. Vinken and G. W. Bruyn (eds.), Handbook of Clinical Neurology, Vol. 15. Elsevier-North Holland Publishing Co. Inc., New York.
Reynolds, E. H. 1975. Chronic antiepileptic toxicity: A review. Epilepsia 16: 319-352.
Richens, A. 1976. Drug Treatment of Epilepsy. Year Book Medical Publishers Inc., Chicago. 176 pp.

Intoxication

Diamond, W. D., and R. A. Buchanan. 1970. A clinical study of the effect of phenobarbital on diphenylhydantoin plasma levels. J. Clin. Pharmacol. 10:306-311.

Kutt, H. 1975. Interactions of antiepileptic drugs. Epilepsia 16:393-402.
Plaa, G. L. 1975. Acute toxicity of antiepileptic drugs. Epilepsia 16:183-191.

Allergy

Livingston, S. L., L. L. Pauli, and I. Pruce. 1978. No proven relationship of carbamazepine therapy and blood dyscrasias. Letter to Ed. Neurology 28:101.
Silverman, S. H., D. Gribetz, and A. R. Rausen. 1978. Nephrotic syndrome associated with ethosuccimide. Am. J. Dis. Child. 132:99.

Idiosyncracy

Ambrosetto, G., C. A. Tassinari, A. Baruzzi, and F. Lugarcsi. 1977. Phenytoin encephalopathy as probable idiosyncratic reaction: Case report. Epilepsia 18:405-408.
Booker, H. E. 1975. Idiosyncratic reactions to the antiepileptic drugs. Epilepsia 16:171-181.
Borgstedt, A. D., M. F. Bryson, L. W. Young, and G. B. Forbes. 1972. Long-term administration of antiepileptic drugs and the development of rickets. J. Pediatr. 81:9-15.
Dent, C. E., A. Richens, D. J. F. Rowe, and T. C. B. Stamp. 1970. Osteomalacia with long term anticonvulsant therapy in epilepsy. Brit. Med. J. 4:69-72.
Luhdorf, K., and M. Lund. 1977. Phenytoin-induced hyperkinesia. Epilepsia 18:409-415.
Richens, A., and D. J. F. Rowe. 1970. Disturbance of calcium metabolism by anticonvulsant drugs. Brit. Med. J. 4:73-76.
Stores, G. 1975. Behavioral effects of antiepileptic drugs. Dev. Med. Child Neurol. 17:647-658.

Malformations

DeVore, G. R., and D. M. Woodbury. 1977. Phenytoin: An evaluation of several potential teratogenic mechanisms. Epilepsia 18:387-396.
Feldman, G. L., D. D. Weaver, and E. W. Lourien. 1977. The fetal trimethadione syndrome. Am. J. Dis. Child. 131:1389-1392.
Janz, D. 1975. The teratogenic risk of antiepileptic drugs. Epilepsia 16:159-169.
Rosen, R. C., and E. S. Lightner. 1978. Phenotypic malformation in association with maternal trimethadione therapy. J. Pediatr. 92:240-244.
Smith, D. W. 1977. Teratogenicity of anticonvulsant drugs. Am. J. Dis. Child. 131:1337-1339.

11
OTHER APPROACHES TO SEIZURE MANAGEMENT

There are numerous other effective methods of seizure control besides just giving medicines. Sometimes these approaches can be used instead of a drug; sometimes they improve the control achieved by the medication. The major approaches are: 1) managing the stresses of common life experiences, 2) behavioral management, 3) neurosurgical approaches, and 4) developing approaches, often using experimental devices. There are other approaches under consideration that have not proven beneficial.

MANAGING COMMON STRESSES OF LIFE

Certain common stresses of life may bring on a seizure or may aggravate a seizure tendency. These stresses include: 1) alcohol and drug usage, 2) allergies, 3) foods and fluids, including special diets and constipation concerns, 4) menstruation and pregnancy, 5) sleep extremes, and 6) trauma.

Alcohol and Drug Intake

Alcohol and drugs (both prescribed and illegal drug usage) may aggravate a seizure problem or may produce one. In general it is best to avoid these substances.

Alcohol can bring out or create a seizure problem that may persist even if the alcohol is discontinued. The greater danger of seizures occurs when the patient is recovering from the state of intoxication. Alcoholism, like drug usage, is a growing problem in children and must be considered in the pediatric age group as well as in the adult population. A related difficulty is that an epileptic patient may appear drunk, either because of a seizure attack or because of too much medication, and he may be mistaken for an alcoholic, especially if there is a record of alcoholism in the patient or his associates.

Illegal drugs have been considered by some as possibly alternate methods of treating seizures. However, observations suggest that these drugs are more likely to aggravate than to help seizures, especially in the drug withdrawal period. Marijuana is suspected to increase susceptibility to seizures. Animal experiments have determined that LSD probably has this same tendency. The patient and his family should be counseled about this possibility. Such drugs are best avoided.

Prescribed drugs, especially tranquilizers, stimulants, and antidepressant medications used in psychiatric problems, may aggravate seizure problems. Some patients have seizures only when on these medications, which may alter the blood levels of anticonvulsants or directly alter the brain functions, allowing a seizure breakthrough. Many times an alternative approach through direct behavioral intervention is more desirable. The drug may serve as a temporary means of beginning such therapy, or at times as a convenient substitute. Sedative drugs and anticonvulsants can also do this. In a seizure patient, these "psychiatric drugs" and sedatives should be avoided if at all possible; however, if necessary, either the patient and his family should be counseled about the possibility of a seizure reaction or the patient should be protected with an ongoing safe anticonvulsant.

Allergies

Allergies do not cause seizures. They may aggravate a seizure problem, as may the medications used to overcome the allergy symptoms. If such a relationship is noted, seeking help in the management of the allergic problem may benefit the patient's general functioning as well as his seizure control. Hints of an allergic component may be the seasonal accentuation of a seizure problem or breakthroughs occurring in certain environments.

Food and Fluids

Skipping meals, excesses or deficiencies of certain food substances, or an overly abundant intake of fluids may aggravate the seizure tendency. Special diets may be an alternative treatment method with some patients.

Regularity Some individuals are sensitive to missing meals. Younger children may experience abnormally low blood sugar levels in the morning. If breakfast is delayed or missed, the child may seize. Regular meals and balanced diets are desirable for seizure patients of all ages.

Special Diets For some individuals the usual diet may include substances that trigger allergic reactions or that cannot be metabolized normally by the body. It is desirable, although not always possible, to identify the problem before trying to overcome it through a special diet. Once the problem is identified, altering the choice of foods to provide any substances lacking by the body but to avoid any substances that the body cannot tolerate may help to lessen the seizure problem.

Some food substances may lead to a drop in the blood sugar level; other substances may produce a rise in the ammonia levels in the blood; still other substances may result in an accumulation of some irritating breakdown products but not result in the needed final products of metabolism. Identification of the problem, and, whenever possible, overcoming it, may not only improve seizure control but also prevent further damage.

Some children may need more than the usual requirements of vitamin B_6 (pyridoxine) in their diet, either because of an inborn metabolic error increasing the requirements for pyridoxine or because of a deficiency in the diet. Sometimes the use of certain medicines (e.g., drugs that fight tuberculosis) lowers the available supply of pyridoxine. Young infants may have been deprived of the vitamin during gestation. In the past, improper preparation of commercial milk accounted for pyridoxine deficiency, but this problem no longer exists. The patient may present with anemia, seizures, and other neurologic handicaps in early life. A trial of high-dosage pyridoxine is not harmful and may be strikingly helpful.

Anticonvulsants may lead to a deficiency in vitamin D_3 or folic acid, which may result in disturbances of bone formation and calcium metabolism or a peculiar anemia with large red blood cells. The pregnant patient or a newborn baby may be especially prone to megaloblastic anemia, and the seizure patient should be watched for this. If any such symptoms are discovered, by observation or by laboratory screening, the lacking vitamin should be supplemented. However, excessive folic acid, especially if not clinically necessary, may decrease seizure control.

At times families may feel that special diets, dietary supplements, or other activities may be useful in improving seizure control. Since these approaches are not potentially harmful, it is probably wiser to allow the patient to try these measures. The family may be more cooperative if the physician concurs with these efforts, but an agreement should be made that these measures constitute an addition to, not a replacement for, medical therapy. If the approach works, the patient has benefited — and the physician may learn something.

Ketogenic Diet In the younger child for whom anticonvulsants have not been effective in controlling the seizures or have not been tolerated, a ketogenic diet may be tried. The diet is a rather unpleasant approach in which the majority of the daily caloric intake is obtained from fatty foods rather than from foods high in carbohydrates, the latter being the normal major component of a meal. This high-fat diet is difficult to make and to maintain. The taste is so bad that the patient may not tolerate or accept it. The excessive fats produce chemicals in the system that are called ketones. Ketones can and must be measured in the urine by dipping a special strip of chemically treated paper into a urine sample or by placing a drop of urine on special diagnostic pills. If ketones are present, meaning that the desired state is obtained, there is a distinct color change in the test paper or pill. A variant on this diet uses medium chain triglyceride fatty substances as the main source of the fats. This diet is easier to prepare, tastes better, and has less restriction on the intake of carbohydrates.

The ketogenic diet seems most effective in the preschool or early school-age child; it seldom works after 8 years of age. Seizures most responsive to it include the myoclonic, akinetic, and atypical absence seizures. Sometimes it is useful with generalized motor seizures, seldom with typical absence seizures, and rarely with psychomotor attacks. If the diet is effective, the initial response may be striking.

One problem with this diet is that there is a tendency for the diet to become less effective. Another problem is that parents may not persist in maintaining the detested diet. A break in the diet may result in the rapid disappearance of ketosis and recurrence of seizures within hours. The diet may be accidentally broken if the physician prescribes a medicine that contains a sugar base, as is often true of liquid medications.

Often the patient is hospitalized at the introduction of the diet. The purpose of the hospitalization is to monitor the degree and onset of the ketotic state and to watch out for significant drops in blood sugar, which may occur for the first few weeks, especially in the morning. The diet may be begun by starving the patient for a few days. The patient is then changed from a high-carbohydrate, low-fat diet to the reverse (low-carbohydrate, high-fat) by stages over a few days. Because this high-fat diet does not contain all nutritional elements needed, the patient is put on preparations containing iron and calcium and on a multiple vitamin preparation containing both the B-complex and D vitamins. Extra care must be taken to see that the patient gets enough protein for growth. The proper state of ketosis is reached when the patient constantly shows ketones on the urine test. The family and the patient must be trained to test the urine at home.

The taste and type of the diet may cause the patient to refuse the food, to vomit, or to experience nausea or stomach cramps. Occasionally the supplements to the diet produce constipation. The family may object to the special food preparation, the effort needed to get the child to eat the food, or the urine monitoring. In the initial stages, excessive drowsiness, low blood sugar levels, and GI complaints may occur. Screening to be sure that the patient does not have a metabolic disturbance in which ketosis is produced by missing meals, resulting in low blood sugar levels, may be valuable; if such a disturbance is found, the ketogenic diet still may be used, but with more caution. Other potential complications include the development of kidney stones, and, if the diet is chronically used, retardation of growth. The diet also may raise the blood levels of some of the anticonvulsant drugs. If the patient is on Diamox, and especially if he also develops an infection, there may be an excessive accumulation of acid in the body.

Another concern is that the high-fat diet may lead to the development of atherosclerosis later in life. It may be wise to check the patient's blood and the family history for any tendency toward high fat content in the blood and early atherosclerotic vascular problems.

The ketogenic diet may be effective, but its effectiveness may not persist, especially if the state of ketosis is not strictly maintained. When it seems desirable to do so, the diet can be discontinued by the gradual re-introduction of the more familiar foods.

Constipation Seizure patients seem more prone to have constipation. This tendency may be attributable to the medications or dietary and fluid management, possibly to the seizures, or to underlying neurologic handicaps. Constipation may be found after the patient has had a seizure; this does not mean that the constipation is the cause of the seizure — it is not. Usually it is best to treat the constipation conservatively by dietary manipulation or by mild laxatives. Enemas, when necessary, should be used infrequently, as should the more potent laxatives. Frequent laxative use may encourage the tendency toward constipation, although it may temporarily relieve the problem.

Fluids Drinking an excess of fluids may aggravate a seizure tendency. In rare cases, marked fluid intake may produce convulsions. This tendency is especially seen around the time of menstrual periods. The fluid intake should be limited to a low normal intake or even a slightly reduced intake in patients who seem exceptionally sensitive. Reduced fluid intake is most useful to patients with generalized seizures, although it may also be useful to patients with absence attacks and with flickering light sensitivity. If such an approach is used, adjustments must be made for fevers, vomiting or diarrhea, excessive sweating, or exceptionally hot environments.

Menstrual Periods and Pregnancy Young women may have a worse seizure problem just before, during, or right after a menstrual period. This problem may be controlled during the seizure-prone period by reducing salt and fluid intake or by giving ammonium chloride, or by using Diamox either during the anticipated time or as an ongoing medication if the periods cannot be anticipated accurately. Some anticonvulsant drugs may be elevated slightly in preparation for each period, but not to the point of intoxication.

In light of the risk for malformations in their children, it may be wiser for epileptic women to avoid pregnancy. If a pregnancy is planned, an effort may be made to taper off the medication prior to conception. However, if this is not possible because of the need for the medication to control the seizures, the patient should be made fully aware of the risks and the medications chosen should be those that have the least risk but are effective. These drugs must be monitored closely and carefully during the pregnancy so as to avoid any intoxication or anemia.

Pregnancy itself tends to bring out brainwave abnormalities. Some women have seizures only when they are pregnant, some experience the onset of a persistent seizure problem with pregnancy, some experience an increase of their seizure frequency with pregnancy, and a rare individual notes improvement of her seizures when she is pregnant.

True gestation seizures are those seizures that occur only at the time of pregnancy and are not related to toxemic complication of the pregnancy. A patient with high blood pressure, protein in the urine, and excessive weight gain who retains fluids in her body may have seizures as a complication of her toxemia. True gestation seizures tend to be focal and often do not recur during the pregnancy, although they may sometimes occur in some but not all succeeding pregnancies. The evaluation is the same as with any other new seizure problem. Whether or not the patient treats the first seizure or waits for a recurrence depends on the severity of the problem, the diagnostic findings, and the personal opinions of the physician and patient.

Status epilepticus is rare during pregnancy unless there is a definite reason. In the past the therapy was to give anticonvulsants and to end the pregnancy, often while the patient was on strong medical management. Both the mother and the offspring had problems. Now efforts are made to control the seizure with vigorous anticonvulsant therapy, often allowing the pregnancy to continue to its completion. The exception to this is when the seizures are due to toxemia, for which the therapy often must be delivery of the infant.

With pregnancy the patient or the physician may make added efforts to control seizures with more diligent intake of the anticonvulsants, rather than risk any problems to either the mother or offspring. On the other hand, the fear of a malformation in the unborn child or problems with vomiting may reduce the medicine intake. Drops in the blood levels of anticonvulsants may be due to increased body metabolism produced by the pregnancy, to related problems of slowed GI movements interfering with drug absorption, to excessive weight gains, or to pregnancy shifts of body fluids. Water and chemical shifts, hormonal changes and the emotional stresses of pregnancy may directly stimulate the brain to seize. Probably the seizure problems of pregnancy are the result of multiple factors.

Unless it is exceptionally severe or prolonged, a seizure is not felt to be dangerous to the mother or to the unborn child, the primary risks being problems of blood circulation and of getting enough oxygen to the placenta or the vigor of the movements. It is now being considered that the anticonvulsants, certain drugs more than others, may be more risky than the seizures. A pregnant woman should be closely monitored, with the evaluations including frequent blood counts and measurements of anticonvulsant levels. Monitoring should be at least monthly. Folic acid may be supplemented either as a separate entity or as part of a multivitamin preparation, especially if an anemia begins to appear. Excessive weight gain or fluid retention should be avoided. The anticonvulsant blood levels must never be allowed to rise above normal and indeed may be best kept in the mid to lower therapeutic range if possible.

Sleep: Too Much or Too Little

Non-alertness, drowsiness, or light sleep (as in falling asleep or in awakening) is a time in which some seizures are most apt to occur. This is especially true with psychomotor attacks, myoclonic seizures, and atypical absence spells. Since a normal sleep pattern cycles from deep to light sleep states, seizures may relate to these cycles during the night as well as during daytime naps. People who experience seizures only at night with sleep (nocturnal seizures) for the first few years of their seizure problem are often unlikely to experience a daytime attack. They may experience few restrictions on employment and driving, and very few restrictions during the daytime. Most seizures that occur during sleep as well as during the daytime wakening hours are but sleep-altered variations of the same seizure problem. Unlike purely nocturnal seizures, which are limited to the sleep state, the latter group are a nighttime accentuation of a seizure problem.

Sometimes the tendency toward seizures in sleep may be reduced by increasing the evening dosage of anticonvulsant medication. If the seizures occur with falling asleep in the early evening, the supper dosage may be increased; if they tend to occur in the early morning around the time of awakening, the approach may be to increase the bedtime dosage of medication or to use a longer-acting anticonvulsant or a time-release capsule.

It has been suggested in the past that sleeping with the light on and with a ticking clock or radio in the room may also decrease the tendency toward seizing. This is at least worth a trial.

Regular sleep habits are important, especially to those with sleep-related seizures. Seizures may be triggered by missing sleep or sometimes even by getting too much sleep. Some people who cannot fall asleep may use sedatives that tend to aggravate the seizure problem. They may be drowsy the next day, which itself aggravates the seizure tendency. They may resort to coffee or stimulant medications to overcome the drowsiness, a practice that can exacerbate some seizures, especially if the stimulating substance is used in excess. Problems in falling asleep may be overcome by increasing the evening medication, by avoiding the use of stimulating substances, especially in the late afternoon or evening, by calm evening activities, or by using a mild bedtime sedative and behavioral training to establish a more efficient sleep pattern.

Drowsiness will almost certainly increase daytime seizures. Sometimes stimulants and caffeine-containing substances given early in the day may be used to increase alertness and to overcome the seizure-provoking tendency if the substances themselves do not trigger seizures or do not excessively interfere with the absorption of the anticonvulsants. Behavioral training approaches may be used to maintain optimum alertness during the day as well as to interrupt some of the seizures that do break through.

Trauma Protection

Some individuals have a seizure only as an immediate consequence to hitting their heads, and some have seizures as a sequel to head trauma. For those who seize whenever they suffer a blow to the head, ongoing anticonvulsive protection may lessen this tendency.

When a significant blow to the head occurs, even if it does not produce a fracture or major injury, the victim may experience a seizure immediately or soon afterward, or within weeks, within months, or even years later. The young child is more prone to convulse than the adult. More severe head injuries are much more apt to result in seizures than minor ones. Sometimes a blow to the head is the result of an unrecognized first seizure and the identified seizure is really a recurrence... thus the head trauma is a result, not a cause, of the seizure.

Immediate seizures are probably related to the stunning of and shock to the brain, with a consequent disruption of function. Early seizures may be due to the irregular effect of the shock or recovery, to irritation from bleeding or a fracture, or to the oversensitivity of the recovering brain cells. Later seizures are probably due to scars from brain damage.

There are certain factors that tend to predict the chances or risks of a later seizure problem but there is no absolute indicator. If the blow produces a prolonged period of unconsciousness, if it produces a fracture with a portion of the bone pressed into or against the brain surface, or if the traumatic object penetrates through the brain coverings, the patient is at greater risk for later seizures. Focal or abnormal neurologic findings, especially if they persist, are also high-risk factors. If there is a significant interval of months or especially of years between the original trauma and the onset of the seizures, the persistence of seizures becomes relatively greater. The longer the duration of the active seizure problem is, the less likely the patient is to overcome the need for active anticonvulsant controls. Some physicians will place patients on one or two anticonvulsants after the trauma in order to prevent a seizure from developing; others will wait for the seizure to occur before initiating therapy. The choice may well be based on the risks for development of a seizure disorder and the risks to the patient should he have a seizure, particularly when he is in the state of recovery from the trauma. It is wiser to begin one drug at a time and to use the safest drugs, avoiding oversedation, which might mask vital observations if the patient is unconscious.

Some seizure patients fall or are flung down with such force by their seizures that they experience severe and repeated head trauma. They may have a history of facial cuts, skull fractures, damage to the teeth, and assorted bruises and bleeds. Those working or living with the patient have a fairly realistic concern regarding the possibility of additional damage to the brain from the seizures. However, there is the tendency to over-restrict the patient in needed activities, including schooling and training experiences. This merely exchanges one handicap for another. While efforts are being made by the physician to overcome the seizures through more effective management, the patient may be protected by use of a special helmet. This head gear may or not include a face guard. Suitable helmets may be obtained from the local sporting goods store from the collection of hockey, football, boxing, or kayak helmets. These are often hard plastic shells with a soft protective inner lining. They are heavy and bulky, but effective. Softer and lighter helmets, such as those obtainable from DanMar Products, Incorporated, of Ann Arbor, Michigan, are lighter, less awkward, washable, and often more acceptable because they are less hot; even though they are also less protective, these lighter helmets are often quite satisfactory. Use of the helmet may allow the patient to return to needed training or educational activities as well as free the parents from worry and consequent overprotection.

BEHAVIORAL APPROACHES

Behavioral approaches not only can be most effective with the consequences of the seizures but also in some cases they may be the primary approach toward controlling the attacks. The behaviorist, be he a psychiatrist, a psychologist, or someone knowledgeable in behavioral techniques and gifted with good observational powers and common sense, is a valuable member of an epilepsy team. The major areas of behavioral intervention include counseling, crisis intervention, helping with coping, and behavior modification, which can be used as a direct intervention with seizures.

Counseling and Misconceptions (See also Chapter 12)

The seizure patient deals with two problems, his self-image and the seizure responsibility. The patient, especially if he is an adolescent, asks himself three basic questions in developing his self-image: Who am I? What am I doing now? Where am I going? The answers may be undesirable and discouraging to the epileptic patient, which may result in surrender or in denial. The response can result in bad habits and irregularities in seizure care, which aggravate the seizure management.

Often there is a conflict between the patient and the parent about "ownership of the seizures." The parent acts as if the seizures are his concern and his responsibility; the patient, especially an adolescent, often goes along with this. The result is an overprotective parent who tends to nag the child about seizure management and a child who acknowledges that the seizures are the parent's problem, not his. The child takes no responsibility for the seizures, the medication, or monitoring attacks. He may not even know what medications he is on. The other extreme is the child who rebels against the overprotective parent either by denying the seizure problem and thus not cooperating in the seizure care or else by using the threat of a seizure in a manipulative manner to obtain his own desires from the parents.

Counseling A person working with the epileptic patient should attempt to understand these two problems through the patient's viewpoint; if he can achieve this, not only may he better understand the patient and the patient's needs, but also he may be able to promote better understanding in the family, the school, and in others. Efforts should be made to shift the direct responsibility for seizure care from the parent to the child as soon as the child is capable. The role of the family and others should be to be a resource. The seizure problem belongs to the patient, but those around him should be willing to help him. Efforts should be made to improve the patient's self-image and to offer more hope and a better future than the patient may believe possible. Overcoming these two problems may result in better control because the patient is now involved.

Group Therapy Gathering together seizure patients, families, or parents may be most effective. Suddenly the individual finds that he is not the only one with the same problem. Sharing experiences, struggles, and solutions may open up more hope. In a clinic, hospital, training program, or school, sometimes a patient or parent may be more effective as a counselor than the trained expert. Patients also may be very effective teachers in a formal teaching presentation, whether it be to clients, to the public, or to professionals. Group therapy, whether at a formal psychologic meeting or as an informal get-together (as with some of the advocacy groups, such as the local chapters of the Epilepsy Foundation of America) often can generate ideas on how to manage various problems that experts have overlooked. Out of these sessions may come alternative ideas, more practical approaches, and suggestions that common methods may not work the best. These offer an opportunity to express frustrations to an understanding and accepting group. The members may grow to support each other. Sometimes more changes can be accomplished by such a group working together than by a single individual in a community.

Coping with the Consequences of Epilepsy (See Chapters 12–14)

Mistaken management of seizure-related problems, although well-meaning, may often be more harmful than helpful. More often, seizure-related problems are overlooked, and total dependence is put on the pills. No single discipline is expert in all aspects of epilepsy. The secret of successful counseling in coping with epilepsy and its consequences is the team approach, which involves diverse experts working together. The rewards often are not just an overcoming of the consequences but an improvement in the seizure control, for the patient is less distracted by having to deal with the other problems and is more cooperative in working toward seizure management. He realizes that the team treats him as a person, not as a seizure disorder.

Crisis Intervention

The seizures and their consequences often explode into the patient's life and the family activities as a catastrophe, resulting in a series of crises, both real and imagined. The two approaches in managing these are in preparation and education of the patient and his family in the handling of these problems as they occur and in the availability of the physician or pertinent team member when a crisis occurs. Preparation and availability of help often reduce mountains to molehills.

Behavioral Management of Seizures

For centuries various behavioral techniques were practiced in seizure control. Sometimes these proved to be very effective. With the advent of the discovery of the anticonvulsant drugs and surgical techniques, total dependence is now placed on drugs and surgery, with behavioral techniques often forgotten or ridiculed as "mysticism." Yet some respected centers are making much use of behavioral approaches, not just for management of the consequences of the seizures but as methods of direct seizure control, sometimes even as an alternative to medication. With some patients the results are impressive.

Behavioral controls imply using various methods to manipulate the environment in order to modify certain seizure-related behaviors and thus to improve seizure control. For example, efforts may be aimed at halting or interfering with the development of a seizure at an early stage of an attack, or even altering environmental activities to prevent the patient's seizure reaction to his surroundings. The first consideration therefore is that the seizure is part of a chain of related events. This allows intervention to become a possibility. The typical chain may be, in sequence: 1) a situational event, 2) a behavioral response, 3) a seizure build-up, 4) the obvious seizure component or event, 5) the reaction of those around the patient, and 6) the response of the patient to these reactions. In some patients the seizure build-up can be subdivided into a series of symptoms in a specific sequence from the initial symptom to the final full attack. For example, roughly a century ago an effective method with focal seizures beginning in the hand and spreading upward was to tie a cloth or rope around the upper arm before the spread reached the elbow. If the tourniquet was applied too late, the seizure often was not halted.

Candidates to be considered for possible behavioral approaches include those with sensory reflex seizures, those who stimulate their own seizures, those with stress-aggravated seizures, and those with seizures related to non-alertness, erratic lifestyles, or a spread from a focal onset. The three main approaches are: 1) altering the patient's reactions to environmental stresses, 2) interrupting the course of a seizure, or 3) modifying the patient's behaviors associated with the attack.

General Considerations Patients who experience disabling, uncontrolled, frequent seizures despite appropriate use of multiple anticonvulsant drugs or in whom surgery is not indicated may be candidates for behavioral approaches. Even patients responding to anticonvulsant drugs or undergoing surgery may find the behavioral methods helpful.

An accurate collection of basic information about the patient, his environment, and his seizures is important. A detailed interview with the family and others who are involved may create a positive attitude toward cooperative efforts. It is important to learn the goals and expectations of the patient and his family. It is equally important to be sure that other members of the total team of people working with patients (physicians, nurses, behaviorist, family, school, etc.) are aware of and in agreement with the goals and aims of the approach, and that consistent use of the methods is developed. The neurologist should stabilize the anticonvulsants in the safe therapeutic range and be willing then to forgo any major changes unless absolutely necessary so that the effect of the behavioral approaches can be judged.

The seizures must be considered both by direct observation and by interviewing the parents and teachers to gain their observations. This involves searching for potentially alterable behaviors that precede or are part of the early stages of the attack. Noting events in the environment that might have triggered the attack is essential. Verifying the relationship of these events to the attacks then must be done, possibly by subjecting the patient to the same stimulation while an EEG is being performed. Noting the state of alertness at the time of the attacks is most useful. Any event that relates to the occurrence of a seizure should be considered.

After a good picture of the step-by-step events of the seizures, their frequency, and possible potentiating events has been obtained, and the information from a good neurologic and psychologic evaluation is reviewed, the picture becomes clearer. Seizure-associated behavior disorders also may be noted. A plan for management is then developed. Based on the team's opinions, the patient's hopes, and the family's expectations, a reasonable set of goals is established. Then a management approach is chosen, including specific methods, a reinforcement schedule, and a clear indication of what behaviors are to be rewarded, what is to be tolerated, what is to be ignored, and what is to be "punished."

Utilizing the recognized patterns and the self-control potentials of the patient combined with strategies developed to alter or suppress the seizures, the patient, the family, and others are trained in activities that decrease the undesirable behaviors (such as seizures) or promote normal behaviors (such as not having seizures). This training must be reinforced by a reward or by a punishment. After a specific interval of time, the responses should be reviewed, comparing the seizure frequency and severity measured for a period prior to the use of the behavioral control methods to the frequency after a set period of use of these methods.

The evaluator must consider the normal tendencies of seizures to wax and wane in frequency. Is the therapy specifically designed to alter the seizure frequency any more effective than a supposedly ineffective method that the patient or family believes will stop the seizure (i.e., a placebo)? Is the improvement significant? Will it be as effective in the normal environment of home, school, or employment as it was in the hospital environment? Will the effect persist?

Situations and Specific States There are some situations and some environmental states that are apt to produce seizures in certain patients. Anxiety-producing situations or environments filled with flashing lights or other rhythmic sensations to which the patient is overly sensitive should be avoided. This is not always possible. The alternative would be to attempt to protect the patient against the overwhelming effects of these influences as well as to work with him to build up his tolerance to these factors. Using sunglasses or colored lenses, avoiding sharp contrasts and a darkened room when watching television, sitting in front of and reasonably far enough back from a movie screen or television set, rather than close or to the side, and avoiding looking at the screen when the picture goes bad and rolls may greatly reduce the chances of precipitating a seizure in a photosensitive patient. Anxiety-provoking or overly exciting events may be handled by preparing the patient for the event through counseling and, if needed, by giving a dosage of Valium prior to the actual event. These are often useful techniques but the obvious desired approach is to train the patient to cope with the stimuli without having a seizure.

The state of alertness is most important. Boredom, prolonged activity, or being ignored may allow the patient to drift into a drowsy state in which such attacks as atypical absences may occur. Sometimes even after a seizure has begun it may be interrupted by calling the person's name or by a loud sound, strong odor, pinch, or pinprick, if not by a mere touch or other unexpected sensory stimulation. The effect that such stimulation has may mean that the seizure is mistaken for a hysterical attack, when indeed such a "recall" phenomenon is seen with seizures. Obviously, establishing regular and adequate sleep habits and strict avoidance of overmedication are most important. However, these measures may not be enough. Involving the patient in briefer and hopefully more stimulating activities that hold his interest will help to keep him alert. Frequent changes in activities may be helpful. Whenever the patient appears to be uninterested, bored, or inattentive, the parent or teacher should call to him or otherwise stimulate him back to full alertness. Ultimately it is desirable to teach the patient to monitor and maintain his own alertness by applying similar techniques, especially when he feels his mind beginning to wander.

Interruption Noting the sequence of the seizure symptoms is most important. An effort is then made to interrupt this sequence before the full seizure emerges. This not only involves interrupting the seizure sequence but often includes reinforcement techniques that encourage behaviors that seem to prevent seizures. Preventing a child from seeking out a bright light or waving his hands before his eyes to create a triggering sensation if this leads to a light-sensitive reflex convulsion is an example of preventive interruption, i.e., preventing the seizures by interrupting the behaviors that lead to the seizure reaction. A sharp vocal command — "No!" — while applying a gentle physical restraint on the hand, arm, or head movements that seem to produce the attack, as with hand-waving motions, may be effective. In seizure attacks that begin with a posturing or a limb movement, replacing the limb in the normal position, followed within a few seconds by a reinforcing reward or punishment, may stop the seizure and lessen future attacks. Introducing a strong sensory stimulation may halt an actual seizure attack. When unpleasant stimuli are used (and often these tend to be most effective), the effectiveness relates to the intensity and timing of the stimulation.

Direct Behavior Modification There are essentially three approaches in behavior management: reward management, developing self-controls, and formal psychologic approaches.

Reward management can be by six methods: 1) *Denial of reward* means withholding a reward whenever an undesirable behavior, such as a seizure, occurs. This may consist of ignoring a seizure rather than giving any attention or displaying an excess of care and concern. 2) A *penalty program* involves withholding a desired privilege or sending the patient out of the room or making him sit in a chair for a brief period of time (i.e., a time-out period) whenever the undesired (seizure) behavior occurs. 3) A *relief* or *avoidance program* gives the patient a chance to avoid an unpleasant experience as a reward for reducing the frequency of the seizures. 4) A *punishment program* results in some form of punishment being administered to the patient whenever undesirable behavior or an increase in seizures occurs. 5) An *overt reward program* is the giving of a specific reward, mutually agreed upon, whenever a set goal is reached, such as a determined lower number of seizures. 6) A *covert reward program,* rather than having the patient earn merits or tokens redeemable for an object or an activity as a reward, involves the psychologist working with the patient's imagination to create the feeling of satisfaction and approval when seizures do not occur, as compared to the unpleasant negative feelings when seizures are common.

The patient may be trained in various types of self-control. He may notice that certain behaviors or actions seem to improve, if not entirely control, his seizures. If this appears possible, his approach and efforts should be encouraged. Helping the patient to relax when he feels stressed or whenever he feels a seizure coming on may be effective, especially when anxiety is a prominent factor. Desensitization approaches also are very useful. The patient is gradually helped to cope with stresses and anxieties, beginning with small, safe exposures. As he proves able to tolerate the small stresses, gradually more stressful situations are introduced at a rate the patient can tolerate, until he can tolerate the major stresses as well as the minor ones. Traditional psychotherapy may be a valuable approach both in crisis intervention and in the development of coping mechanisms. In the one-to-one situation, the patient must be helped to understand his problem and to develop and apply appropriate methods of handling the seizure-producing conflicts and anxieties.

Psychophysiologic Approaches Two approaches commonly used are 1) conditioning, habituation, or extinction approaches in developing tolerances to a seizure-producing sensation and 2) biofeedback. In conditioning approaches, a sensory stimulus shown to trigger seizures is given repeatedly until it no longer produces the attacks. The stimulus can be given in one or both eyes, ears, or body sides. Often the stimulus may be begun at a low intensity and frequency and as a presentation similar but not identical to the triggering pattern. As the patient tolerates this, the stimulation is made more and more like the offending stimuli until the patient can tolerate even the primary precipitating pattern without having a seizure. For example, the patient may have a few EEG leads applied and connected to a flashing light. The light is turned on to a frequency beneath but close to that to which the patient is sensitive. As he tolerates this, the frequency is raised by small stages closer and closer to the previously intolerable flash frequency. Whenever abnormal bursts appear on the EEG, the flashing light is stopped until the EEG normalizes; then it begins again. This is practiced daily until the patient tolerates flashing lights at all frequencies without any abnormal reactions. Strict efforts are made to prevent any seizure reaction by not allowing the light to persist the moment that the EEG shows the abnormal activities. Similar approaches can be applied to any sensory reflex seizures. Unfortunately, the developed tolerance may not persist. Efforts are now being developed to provide reinforcing reminders to maintain the protection through the use of specific devices.

Biofeedback has been tried with seizures as with other physiologic reactions, such as migraines. Unfortunately it has not yet proven effective. In biofeedback, the patient is trained to recognize abnormal EEG patterns during recording sessions. Sometimes the brainwave abnormalities are also translated into a click or a similar sensory stimulation to assist the patient's recognition. He is trained to concentrate on producing good waves and stopping bad ones. Some approaches use a variant in which the abnormal brainwaves will trigger an unpleasant reward, such as a shock, within a short time unless the patient can avoid it by controlling his own brainwaves through concentration.

Other Methods Other psychologic approaches have been tried. Over-correction, i.e., having the patient repeat a behavioral act similar to but not identical to the act that precipitates a seizure, yet avoiding giving any good rewards, may work. The patient concentrates on the act and is taught to understand the significance of it. He performs it even when it is uncomfortable. For example, the child who waves his hands before his eyes may be required to stand in a corner or sit on a chair and open and close his fists with his arms at his side. This is a method of substituting a different, non-rewarded behavior for an undesired one.

Sometimes efforts are made through behavioral methods to reduce the seizures down to a specific time of day or specific environment. Then intensified medical or psychologic efforts are aimed toward that situation.

Flooding and *implosion* are two behavioral techniques that are used. The patient is repeatedly required to produce the unwanted behavior reaction or response without earning any reward. However, this method can be dangerous: it may tend to trigger seizures rather than reduce their frequency. These approaches may only accentuate the severity and persistence of the problem by training the patient in how to have seizures.

Most often a combination of several methods and approaches is more effective than any single approach used alone.

SURGICAL APPROACHES

Neurosurgical approaches to seizure control may be divided into two situations, necessary relief of a progressive lesion that is causing the seizure (such as a tumor, trauma, or malformation of the brain or blood vessels) or elective surgery as an attempt to control seizures in selected patients when all else has failed.

Elective neurosurgery is directed toward those severely disabled by seizures that have not been adequately controlled despite optimum, intensified, medical and psychological efforts. Seizures most commonly considered for such approaches include temporal lobe epilepsy, focal seizures originating from a relatively non-vital area, and seizures in young children, especially those that are associated with a weakness or paralysis of one side of the body due to severe damage to one-half of the brain. Generalized seizures and multi-focal seizure disorders are essentially not candidates for elective surgery.

Elective Surgery Criteria

Strict criteria have been established so that patients may be selected for surgery who will have a good chance of benefiting from the operation and a low risk for additional problems resulting from surgery. The patient should be reliable, emotionally mature and stable, and fully cooperative; he should have the potential for good functioning provided that the seizure problem can be overcome. The seizure problem must be shown by diagnostic studies and description to be a focal disturbance that can be reached and removed without resultant significant further damage and without unnecessary risks. The seizure problem should have been present for a long enough time (i.e., usually at a minimum of three to five years, and preferably by late adolescence to early adulthood) that the developing seizure will have stabilized rather than still be progressing; the time also should be sufficient to suggest that the seizure problem is persistent and not apt to regress spontaneously. However, with some patients a mirror seizure focus may develop in the opposite brain half in a similar area; if surgery is delayed too long thereafter, the mirror focus may become an independent seizure site and not respond to the surgery, even though the primary focus and its seizure symptoms have been successfully removed. The seizure problem also must be shown to be unresponsive to a full trial of anticonvulsants of various types with monitoring of blood levels to be sure that the doses were adequate. Often the final decision may be made by a team rather than by the neurosurgeon alone. Sometimes when a patient does not fully qualify under the above restrictions, an exception may be made if he has a severe progressive focal seizure problem or he fits into the infantile hemiplegic syndrome.

If the patient is accepted into evaluation, he is then subjected to a full battery of intelligence, language, psychologic, electroencephalographic, and radiologic tests. Evaluation may include obtaining EEG tracings directly from the surface of the brain or from multiple wire electrodes sunk into the brain to strictly localize the size of the seizure focus, as well as air studies, angiograms, and CT scans. Special attempts are made to locate the speech and language centers. One such approach is to place catheter tubes into the arteries on each side of the neck that lead to the brain. With the patient awake and the EEG running, a fast-acting barbiturate is injected into one side, its effect is noted, and then the procedure is repeated on the other side. When the injection is on the side in which language is located, the patient loses his language and speech skills as the EEG shows the effects of the drug. Surgery on the side of language is avoided, or, if necessary, it is approached very conservatively.

Once this information is obtained and reviewed carefully, and if the patient still qualifies, the question is whether the patient will benefit from the operation without acquiring any significant handicap. If the patient is still felt to be acceptable, then this type of approach is considered.

Alternative Surgical Procedures

There are three basic surgical approaches: 1) removing the focal area of the seizure, 2) interrupting the spread of a seizure by various pathways, or 3) removing half of the brain, as is done with the infantile hemiplegic syndrome. A focus may be cut out, frozen, burned out, or destroyed with electricity or radioactivity. The pathways of spread, especially those from one brain half to the other (the corpus callosum), can be severed in the hope of limiting the size of the seizure attacks. In younger children in which one brain half is so damaged that the patient is paralyzed (and often incapacitated in other functions) and has uncontrollable seizures, removing the damaged brain half may not only remove the seizures but may also lead to improvement of the paralysis of the involved side and generally improved functioning. Even the learning and behavior may be improved. Essentially the damaged brain half is beyond any useful function but still discharges the seizure activities that interfere with efforts of the other, relatively good brain half. In light of the much later complications of hydrocephalus and bleeding tendencies, some surgeons resort to a partial removal of the damaged hemisphere, leaving fairly normal tissue and deeper structures behind, in order to reduce these risks.

In the adult these surgical approaches are frequently performed under a local anesthetic, so that the patient can work with the surgeon, reporting any sensations or memories he experiences. The surgeon may stimulate portions of the brain and use the patient's responses to determine where areas of seizure symptoms come from. An EEG can also be used during surgery to help locate potential seizure-causing tissue. Surgery on the brain proper is essentially painless; the only discomfort is on the skin surface and bone coverings, which can be numbed by local anesthesia.

Results

Seizure surgery can be most rewarding in the hands of a conservative team of specialists who practice cautious considerations and a thoughtful screening evaluation as well as conservative surgery. Seizure control and marked seizure improvement occur in a majority of the patients, with a low incidence of new problems and a very low death rate. Often other brain functions may be markedly improved, including even behavior at times.

These surgical techniques don't completely replace the need for anticonvulsants. Often the patient is kept on the medication for a minimum of three to four years of complete control before the medication is gradually discontinued.

OTHER APPROACHES

Researchers are constantly looking for new and better approaches to improved seizure control. Other than needed developments of new drugs, new efforts are being made to develop various reinforcement devices, warning monitors, brain stimulators, and other approaches. These efforts are still largely in the experimental stages of refinement and consequently are not widely available. They must meet rigid government requirements for safety and effectiveness before they can be freely used.

Reinforcement Devices

A major problem with conditioning therapy for sensory reflex seizures is that after the completion of the intensified training period, the effectiveness of the extinction tends to wear off. In an effort to prolong the learned protection, various methods and devices are being developed to remind the subconscious and to reinforce the original training. Essentially, the devices consist of a sensitive receiver that picks up the sensation and translates it into a stimulus that is delivered to the patient to reinforce the previous extinction reaction before the seizure response can occur. Such a device may consist of a photosensitive cell on a glass frame that receives a flash of light and triggers a small light on the inner surface of the glass frame. The patient has been conditioned to regard this small light as a reinforcer that serves as a reminder to the brain not to seize. The audio-stimulator is another such device under development. It looks like a pocket transistor radio with an attached earphone. The unit receives a sound and translates the stimulus to a reinforcing "beep" transmitted to the earphone. The concept is that the "beep" reminds and reinforces the conditioning mechanism not to seize before the sound itself produces the reflex seizure.

Seizure Warning Devices

One instrument under development is a portable monitor, designed to be carried by the patient, which constantly checks the brainwave pattern. When abnormal seizure-like energies begin to build up, the machine automatically warns the patient of the potential seizure breakthrough, thus enabling him to get to a safe place.

Cerebellar and Other Brain Stimulators

Another approach is the development of portable machines that will deliver impulses to wires implanted in various portions of the brain. The goal is to disrupt the build-up and spread of seizure energy within the brain by delivering a counter-stimulation. Usually the patient must sense the impending seizure and trigger the device. Theoretically ideal is the combination of the seizure warning device and the brain stimulator, so that the warning would automatically trigger a counter-stimulation without depending on the patient to respond.

Other Approaches

Acupuncture has been considered for epilepsy. There has been no evidence of its effectiveness. Some people have tried the "consciousness-changing drugs," such as LSD, marijuana, and others, as possible anticonvulsants. Emerging evidence suggests that these drugs may have the opposite effect. Efforts are also being made to isolate various chemicals that carry messages from one nerve cell to another. Some of these increase brain activity and some decrease it. The concept is that methods might be developed to increase the inhibition-transmitting chemicals or to decrease the exciting mediators. Although not successful yet, this idea shows promise.

CONCLUSION

In addition to drugs, there are numerous approaches to effective treatment of epilepsy. Often a combination treatment approach proves to be most effective, especially when it involves a team of experts. The main goal of treatment is to help the patient function at his best potential by using the most conservative therapeutic approach, without subjecting him to any potential risks or actual harm.

REFERENCES AND SUGGESTED READING

General

Aird, R. B., and D. M. Woodbury. 1974. The Management of Epilepsy. Charles C Thomas, Springfield, Ill. 448 pp.
Dodson, W. E., A. L. Prensky, D. C. DeVivo, S. Goldring, and P. R. Dodge. 1976. Management of seizure disorders: Selected aspects, Part II. J. Pediatr. 89: 695-703.
Lennox, W. G. 1960. Epilepsy and Related Disorders. Little, Brown & Company, Boston and Toronto. 1168 pp.
Livingston, S. 1972. Comprehensive Management of Epilepsy in Infancy, Childhood, and Adolescence. Charles C Thomas, Springfield, Ill. 657 pp.
Sands, H., and F. C. Minters. 1977. The Epilepsy Fact Book. F. A. Davis Co., Philadelphia. 116 pp.
Solomon, G. E., and F. Plum. 1976. Clinical Management of Seizures. W. B. Saunders Company, Philadelphia. 152 pp.

Life Stresses

Feeny, D. M. 1977. Marijuana and epilepsy. Science 197:1301-1302.
Gordon, N. 1977. Medium-chain triglycerides in a ketogenic diet. Dev. Med. Child. Neurol. 19:535-544.
Knight, A. H., and E. G. Rhind. 1975. Epilepsy and pregnancy: A study of 153 pregnancies in 59 patients. Epilepsia 16:99-110.
Lott, J. T., T. Coulombe, R. V. DiPaolo, E. P. Richardson, Jr., and H. L. Levy. 1978. Vitamin B_6-dependent seizures: Pathology and chemical findings in the brain. Neurology 28:47-54.
Ramsay, R. E., R. G. Strauss, B. J. Wilder, and L. J. Willimore. 1978. Status epilepticus in pregnancy: Effect of phenytoin malabsorption on seizure control. Neurology 28:85-89.

Tassinari, C. A., G. Terzano, G. Capocchi, B. D. Bernardina, F. Vigevana, O. Daniele, C. Valladier, C. Dravet, and J. Roger. 1977. Seizures during sleep. In: J. K. Penry (ed.), Epilepsy, the Eighth International Symposium, pp. 345-354. Raven Press, New York.

Behavioral Approaches

Balashak, B. K. 1976. Teacher implemented behavioral modification in a case of organically based epilepsy. J. Consult. Clin. Psychol. 44:218-223.

Clausen, J. 1977. Psychological intervention with parents of children with seizures. In: J. K. Penry (ed.), Epilepsy, the Eighth International Symposium, pp. 235-238. Raven Press, New York.

Forster, F. M. 1977. Reflex Epilepsy, Behavioral Therapy and Conditional Therapy. Charles C Thomas, Springfield, Ill. 318 pp.

Mostofsky, D. I. 1977. Behavioral therapy for seizure control. In: J. K. Penry (ed.), Epilepsy, the Eighth International Symposium, pp. 239-243. Raven Press, New York.

Mostofsky, D. I., and B. A. Balashak. 1977. Psychobiological control of seizures. Psychol. Bull. 84:723-750.

Zöllner-Breusch, U. 1977. Operant conditioning for behavioral modification in institutionalized retarded children. In: J. K. Penry (ed.), Epilepsy, the Eighth International Symposium, pp. 285-290. Raven Press, New York.

Zultnick, S., W. J. Mayville, and S. Moffat. 1975. Modification of seizure behaviors: The interruption of behavioral chains. J. Appl. Behav. Anal. 8(1):1-12.

Surgical

Falconer, M. A. 1975. The place of surgery in temporal lobe epilepsy in childhood and adolescence. In: H. Narabayashi and P. L. Gildenberg (eds.), Confinia Neurologica, Vol. 37, No. 1-3, Part III. S. Karger, Basel.

Milner, B. 1975. Psychological aspects of focal epilepsy and its neurosurgical management. In: D. P. Purpura, J. K. Penry, and R. D. Walter (eds.), Advances in Neurology, Vol. 8, Chapter 15, pp. 299-321. Raven Press, New York.

Penfield, W., and H. Jasper. 1954. Epilepsy and the Functional Anatomy of the Human Brain. Little, Brown & Company, Boston. 896 pp.

Serafetinides, E. A. 1975. Psychosocial aspects of neurosurgical management of epilepsy. In: D. P. Purpura, J. K. Penry, and R. D. Walter (eds.), Advances in Neurology, Vol. 8, Chapter 15, pp. 323-332. Raven Press, New York.

Talairach, J., and J. Bancaud. 1974. Stereotaxic exploration and therapy in epilepsy. In: O. Magnus and A. M. Lorentz de Haas (eds.), The Epilepsies, Chapter 39, pp. 758-782. P. J. Vinken and G. W. Bruyn (eds.), Handbook of Clinical Neurology, Vol. 15. Elsevier North-Holland Publishing Company, New York.

Walker, A. E. 1974. Surgery for epilepsy. In: O. Magnus and A. M. Lorentz de Haas (eds.), The Epilepsies, Chapter 39, pp. 758-782. P. J. Vinken and G. W. Bruyn (eds.), Handbook of Clinical Neurology, Vol. 15. Elsevier North-Holland Publishing Company, New York.

Experimental

Kaplan, B. J. 1975. Biofeedback in epileptics: Equivocal relationship of reinforced EEG frequency to seizure reduction. Epilepsia 16:477-486 (Comments on above article, 487-495).

12
EMOTIONAL AND BEHAVIORAL CONSEQUENCES OF EPILEPSY

History has swung back and forth between over-emphasizing and denying relationships between emotional problems, behavioral difficulties, and epilepsy. Yet a significant number of patients with seizures are found to have some degree of emotional disturbance, especially if the epilepsy is due to some type of brain damage. There are more problems found than would be expected to occur by chance. Why some patients have major problems, some only minor disturbances, and some no such difficulties remains unclear.

TYPES OF PROBLEMS

Seizure patients may have 1) personality disturbances, 2) anger and aggressive reactions, 3) depressions and suicidal reactions, 4) hysterical behaviors, and 5) psychotic disturbances. Children may have problems of immaturity, hyperactivity, temper, or acting-out episodes.

Causes
It is not known to what degree these problems are directly or indirectly related to the seizure itself or the underlying brain damage, are reactions to the drugs, or are learned responses to the environmental attitudes and distorted self-concepts in the seizure patient. Probably the resultant problems are an interrelated mixture of these factors, varying with each person.

Age Effect
Seizure problems beginning in early childhood are more often associated with personality and character disorders, problems in getting along with

others, aggressive acting-out behaviors, and hyperactivity. Seizures beginning in adolescence or early adulthood are more apt to be associated with depression and discouragement. Patients with a seizure problem of long duration seem to have more emotional and behavior problems than those with seizures of recent onset.

BEHAVIOR PROBLEMS

Behavior problems are more frequent in children than in adults. The child may be less prepared to cope with the stresses of the epilepsy. He is more dependent on others, whose attitudes shape his personality development and social interactions. He may suffer feelings of fear or doom as the early warning sensations of an impending seizure begin to build up. He later awakens, sometimes having wet himself or drooled on his shirt front. He finds himself surrounded by a crowd of shocked, uncomfortable, yet curious onlookers. At the time he may be drowsy and confused, not clearly understanding what is going on or what people are trying to do to him. He may misinterpret what is being said. His ideas and impressions may be distorted and fearful.

As the child grows up, he finds his family to be overly indulgent, overly solicitous, protective, restrictive, or occasionally rejecting of him. He finds that he may not be wanted by other children and other families in the neighborhood, at school, or by society in general. He feels rejected and left out. He soon gets the message that he is different.

The patient is never certain when he will lose control, interrupting his tasks by a seizure, no matter where he is or what he is doing. He finds himself dragged from doctor to doctor, from test to test, and from pill to pill, all aimed at trying to find out what is wrong with him... why he is different. Each doctor tends to talk to the parents before noticing the patient in examining him. Then the physician turns his back again and resumes talking with the parents. The parents may soon become obsessed with giving the medicine at specific times, often nagging the child to do certain things or not to do certain activities that might affect his seizures. The child may adopt these obsessive attitudes or he may rebel against them.

A seizure may be fearful to the younger child. He may fear that he is dying. Sometimes he reacts by publicizing his seizure as if to play down his concerns. The older child is more apt to be embarrassed and ashamed. His seizure is a social catastrophe. Consequently he may try to hide the problem, including the fact that he must take medications. Unfortunately for him, the seizure may not remain hidden. The attitudes of his classmates and teachers contribute to his fears. These anxieties may show up as feelings of shame, disgrace, and ultimate withdrawal from class activities.

With repeated attacks, examinations, and tests, the child often begins to see himself as different and damaged. He tries to adapt to his illness but often his attempts lead to a maladaption. He becomes anxious, fearful, or insecure. He may become very dependent and immature, as if to avoid growing up to face the problems of the seizures. His parents may subconsciously foster this reaction of dependency. Some children rebel against the seizures and the consequent restraints imposed. The adolescent may make this the key point of his adolescent break-away.

Teenagers face a normal adolescent crisis. Basically they seek to answer three major questions: Who am I? What am I doing? Where am I going? That is, they question their identity, abilities, and potentials, and the future. The epileptic teenager may not see hopeful answers. He may see himself as damaged, perhaps incomplete, even possibly grotesque, since often he imagines his attacks to be much worse than they really are. He cannot depend upon himself to function normally because his efforts may be interrupted at any time. His future may seem bleak and limited. The self-concept of the epileptic patient often becomes distorted; frequently, it is very low as compared to that of a non-handicapped individual.

REACTIONS

Disturbed self-concepts produce many emotional conflicts, which emerge as personality distortions and behavioral disturbances. The patient may deny his epilepsy, consequently skipping or stopping his medication. The recurrence of the seizure only reinforces his poor self-concept as his defenses are shattered.

Some patients may become obsessed with taking their medicine and the adherence to a daily routine in order to avoid the attacks. A seizure breakthrough that occurs despite their best efforts can be most discouraging to them.

The child may decide that since the doctor pays attention to, talks with, and explains the problems to the parents, and since the parents are the ones who seem concerned about and nagging about the medications, the seizure problem must be theirs, not his. The older child or adolescent who has this attitude may not even know the strength of, the name of, or the dose schedule for the medicines he is taking. He leaves everything up to his parents. By adolescence, such a reaction may interfere with regular intake of the drugs. The teenager who has not assumed the responsibility for his seizure may be forgetful, manipulative, or rebellious. He is careless in his seizure care because that care is his parents' responsibility, not his. He may rebel against his parents by refusing, omitting, or hiding the medicine in order to punish the parents with a seizure. He may sense his parents' fears and thus use the threat of an attack to manipulate them.

Feelings of inferiority and insecurity may lead to much discouragement. The depressed patient often begins to withdraw from school and any social interactions in which he might be disgraced by a seizure. Sometimes his attitude is marked by negative attitudes toward society, voiced with frank anger. The patient may blame society for not accepting him and his seizure problem. Indeed, often such a patient cannot accept his own seizures. Society is more apt to reject the patient because of his personality than because of his epilepsy. If the depression becomes too great, with the future looking bleak and hopeless, the patient may turn to the prescription of pills as a way out. He may overdose on the medications or he may drive recklessly, as if risking death. Adolescents, young adults, or patients with chronic handicapping seizures are at special risk for such discouragement.

BEHAVIORAL RESPONSES

The child who is overwhelmed by the seizure problem may fear the capricious loss of control, may develop a sense of shame and disgrace, often may feel insecure, and consequently usually develops a damaged self-image. He becomes increasingly anxious about the future. He often becomes irritable, angry, or depressed. In an attempt to cope with these feelings, various disturbances in behavior may emerge.

Withdrawn Defeatist Attitude

The patient may appear shy and secretive, unwilling to participate in activities. He may act dull and dumb in order to avoid attention, decrease demands, and lessen expectations. He feels safer if he is not involved. Such a child needs a supportive explanation and ongoing encouragement with much reassurance.

Rebellious Resentful Attitude

The patient may try to escape, through rebellion, from the smothering, overly restrictive demands placed on him. He may be so discouraged that he lashes out angrily. He may try to blame others for rejecting him because of his epilepsy. He may appear angry, hostile, and aggressive. His school record may be filled with a history of absences. He may develop frank antisocial and delinquent behavior. This child needs intensive guidance and counseling so that he may finally accept his epilepsy and develop a better self-concept and therefore move ahead.

Behavioral Problems

Children struggling with the problem of epilepsy often display acting-out behaviors. They may seem moody or they may display erratic, variable, unpredictable behaviors. Some children seem irritable, exhibiting angry outbursts of temper. Their attention spans may seem shortened. Some children are anxious and jittery, with hyperactive behavior. Understanding, calm counseling, and patient reassurance may be most helpful to them.

Hyperactivity

There are many causes of hyperactivity in children, although the symptoms may be similar. The common denominator of all these causes is that there appears to be some disturbance between the environmental stimuli and the handling of the sensations by the thinking brain. If a clear, balanced flow of these stimuli does not occur, the individual reacts with responses that are called hyperkinetic. The inciting problem may be: 1) a threatening environment with which the child cannot cope, hence resulting in anxiety; 2) a hearing or a visual problem that clouds or distorts incoming stimuli, causing confusion and posing a threat to the child; 3) disturbances in the deeper brain centers that relate to the distribution of the incoming sensations as well as to attention, alertness, and emotions; 4) a learning disability interfering with the early stages of the thinking processes, which are called perception or recognition; 5) placement of the child in a school environment in which he is too bright or of a too low intelligence to be at ease. These children are frustrated, threatened, or overwhelmed, and consequently respond with hyperkinetic behavior.

The hyperactive child may exhibit an excess of impulsive, uncontrolled, unproductive, uninhibited physical activity. He is distractable, inattentive, or short in his attention span. He tends to over-react emotionally, often over-responding to seemingly minor stimuli. He may have trouble getting along with others socially; indeed, he may tease and torment others. Some children do not obey or respond to discipline well. Some children seem too sleepy, but other children seem not to need sleep. A number of hyperkinetic children appear to have specific learning problems, and often the specific learning problem turns out to be the cause, not the result, of the hyperactivity.

In the seizure patient, the environment, the deep brain processes, the early learning stages, and the intelligence all may be causes of hyperkinetic behavior, or the cause may be a mixture of problems, including the environmental stresses. If the problem is primarily environmental, the family often is found to be overly protective and overly indulgent; the child is often spoiled, anxious, and immature. If the child has a learning problem, the hyperactivity may appear primarily in school and homework situations.

If the problem is in the deeper brain areas that help deliver the incoming sensations to vital areas on the brain surface, and which also involve alertness and emotional reactions, three types of personalities may be seen. Some children seem cheerful yet immature. They try, but they cannot control their behavior. They often chatter aloud. They take chances, although their coordination may be poor. Sometimes stimulants, such as Ritalin, Cylert, or Dexedrine, that are part of their therapy, activate seizures in children.

Children with frontal lobe disturbances often seem placid and pleasant but inattentive as they exhibit an aimless, unproductive energy, going from activity to activity. They perseverate, doing the same things over and over again. They do not make social contacts or seem to interact with others. They also may be rather clumsy. The EEG may show a frontal lobe abnormality. A stimulant drug may be of some help but a tranquilizer is apt to over-sedate the child. Behavioral approaches offer the most help.

Although a seizure patient may have any of the above types of hyperkinetic symptoms, he may also have a temporal lobe type of hyperactivity. This may take on more of an aggressive, angry, or destructive nature. The behavior is unpredictable. The child may be difficult to manage. The child with a left temporal lobe seizure problem is more often typically hyperactive, whereas the individual with a right temporal lobe seizure disorder may be more impulsive and aggressive in his reactions. This hyperactivity is especially common when the seizures begin in earlier childhood. Stimulants and tranquilizers are rarely of any benefit and sometimes only aggravate the seizures.

The approach of choice, in terms of long-term benefits, no matter what the cause of the hyperactivity is, consists of counseling and modifying the behaviors. For some selected patients, a stimulant (e.g., Ritalin, Dexedrine, Cylert), or similar medicine may reduce the activities and distractability; it does not affect the long-term outlook: it does not necessarily prevent the child's naturally outgrowing or, alternatively, his growing into delinquency by adolescence. Tranquilizers are temporary measures used to gain control until a more effective approach can be used. They do tend to sacrifice alertness and motivation to learn, and they may aggravate seizures. Dietary manipulations, megadoses of vitamins, and other fads have not proven effective. Any handicap in learning, vision, or hearing should be corrected if treatment is to be effective.

Hysterical Reactions

Some patients discover that their seizures get them out of unpleasant situations or gain them extra attention and benefits. Subconsciously they may imitate seizures that they have seen or they may imitate their own seizures. These attacks become an advantage rather than a liability to them. During an attack, the pupils of their eyes often are not enlarged or are unresponsive to a flashed light — reactions often present in a real major attack. With these patients the best approach may be "benign neglect" and counseling. Pushing anticonvulsants at them may only produce more immature coping skills, leading to an increasing number of seizures. For concomitant real seizures, the anticonvulsants may need to be maintained at a low therapeutic range.

Other Neurotic and Psychotic Reactions

More severe psychiatric problems may emerge with some patients. Although the environmental stresses may be beyond their coping abilities, there is the suggestion that there are also brain factors involved in the emergence of such problems. (Major psychiatric disturbances and minor psychiatric trends are discussed later in this chapter.)

DEPENDENCE VERSUS INDEPENDENCE

Over-indulgent, over-protective, and over-restrictive parents, linked with an insecure, anxious, and discouraged child who has a low self-concept, tend to keep the child immature and dependent. He fears growing up, a fear held in common with his parents. If the attacks remain uncontrolled, the child tends to become more dependent on others for help. The rejecting attitudes of society tend to discourage any attempts toward independence. Part of the adolescent crisis is the struggle between dependence and independence, with the latter being the desired goal. The epileptic child is more handicapped in this struggle. If his seizures are a chronic problem, he may not be able to cope with this struggle; thus he retreats back to dependency. This is especially true if the seizures have been present since early childhood. If the seizures begin during the adolescent period, the patient often is able to make the transition to independence, although the trip may be rough.

This striving toward independence can be encouraged by the patient's family, friends, and physician if they continually stress responsibility and involvement by the seizure patient in his care. The patient should be familiar with the details of his medications and his seizure status. He should assume primary responsibility for his medications, although his parents remain the resource for the purchase of the medications. Responsibility can be encouraged by beginning vocational planning and guidance even in the earlier years with the parents; in the adolescent period this orientation becomes the major thrust.

GENERAL MANAGEMENT

Depending on his age and intelligence, the child should be given as much information about his epilepsy as he is capable of understanding. He should be involved and responsible for remembering to take his medications and report his seizures. He should be checked periodically by interview to see exactly what his understanding and involvement is.

The physician should take care not to neglect the younger patient or turn his back and talk only with the parents. The physician should spend part of his time discussing and explaining pertinent information with the child. The discussion should include talking about the seizure, the tests, the pills, and other therapeutic approaches. (If this discussion is done well, the eavesdropping parents may even understand what the physician is talking about.) Questions and complaints should be encouraged and answered. Indeed, the visit might begin with a brief chat with the child about his seizures and how things are going before the physician turns to the parents to get their full report. The examination should end with a reassuring explanation to the child of what has been determined and what is to be done. Some children are delighted to look at their x-rays, EEG, or CT scan pictures as the doctor explains them. If the physician can make the patient feel important he is more apt to gain his confidence, cooperation, and involvement, as well as the support of the parents.

SEIZURES AND PSYCHIATRIC DISTURBANCES

There is an ongoing debate about whether there is any particular tendency for the seizure patient to have minor and major psychiatric problems. In the past, attempts have been made to identify an epileptic personality as one who is shy, withdrawn, slow, unstable, unpredictable, and rather monotonous and as a person who exhibits widely variable extremes of emotional reactions. In part, such personalities are not uncommon, yet the multiple external pressures, the different types of seizures, and the great variability of the presentation of the seizure problems have given impetus to many doubts about whether a pure "epileptic personality" exists. More likely there are different trends for different patients.

Seizure Types and Behavioral Reactions

Certain seizure types have been associated with behavioral disturbances. The problem may vary according to the location, the side of the brain involved, and the number of years that the seizure problem has been present. More often the emotional and behavioral problems are mild, with no major handicapping or at least no recognized impact on the patient's life. However, these problems may distort the patient's reactions and responses sufficiently to create discontent, frustration, and adjustment problems. The patient may appear emotionally weak, unstable, and self-centered. This is more true with myoclonic epilepsy than with psychomotor epilepsy; it is least often seen with generalized motor attacks. The myoclonic and the psychomotor seizure patients seem to be more vulnerable and less able to cope with life. This may be due to the interactions and effects on the centers of emotion (the limbic system) and the sensory learning areas of the brain surface. Of all seizure patients, the psychomotor seizure patient seems to have the most difficulties in coping. He may be the most difficult patient to rehabilitate. In psychomotor epilepsy, there may be associated significant behaviors and emotional abnormalities seldom seen with other focal seizure disorders.

Responses to Unrecognized Seizure Problems

It is necessary to distinguish between behaviors and emotions that are part of a seizure and those produced by chronic attempts to deal with the problems of epilepsy. Fear or anxiety, but rarely anger, is seen as an initial seizure symptom. This fear must be distinguished from the fear of an impending attack. Feelings of pleasure or of depression may be early symptoms. The depression may persist for a period of time afterward, suggesting that some chemical may be released into the brain as part of the attack.

Some attacks may appear only as a behavioral disturbance. This may not be recognized as such and the patient may be treated as if he were mentally ill or emotionally disturbed. Such management may not only increase the basic behavioral problems already present, but may also result in an increase of the seizures.

Hallucinations and illusions may be seen in both psychotic states and in psychomotor seizures. Seizure hallucinations tend to present as sounds of a musical or mechanical nature, whereas psychotic hallucinations may present as threatening voices. Body distortions or visual hallucinations are seen with psychomotor seizures. Such distortions and visual hallucinations may be quite intense, but, unlike a psychotic hallucination, they tend to be nonthreatening and recognized as unreal. Psychotic hallucinations, by comparison, tend to be threatening and accusatory to the patient.

The Psychomotor (Temporal Lobe) Epilepsy Problem

Some specialists describe a temporal lobe seizure personality and some go so far as to try to specify a "left temporal lobe syndrome" and a "right temporal lobe syndrome." Destructive lesions of the temporal lobe may disrupt the interchange of information between the centers relating to emotions and those relating to sensory learning processes. Seizures may disrupt or overstimulate these centers and their connections. This disruption could result in new and changed associations.

Factors The development of emotional and behavioral problems may relate to the underlying personality, to the age of onset of the seizures, to the location of the disturbance in the brain, to the course of the seizure problem, to the controls over the seizure discharges, to the presence of a lesion or frank brain damage, and to the management of the growing child in general, both at home and at school. Some of these many factors relate primarily to brain function and some to the environment. For example, the child whose psychomotor seizures began before the school years seems more likely to develop such problems as confusion of or forgetting of what he hears, mental retardation, hyperactivity, and rage reactions. It may be that problems in understanding and remembering what is heard underlie the other problems. The parents' reactions to the seizures and to the unrecognized learning difficulties, as well as to the behavioral problems, may aggravate the emerging emotional disturbances and acting-out behaviors. Early intervention, through awareness of these problems and detection of them in the early stages, may help to avoid consequent problems.

The existence of specific personality tendencies relating to specific seizures is controversial. Those arguing against such a relationship note that those in favor of such an association are located in centers that actively work with emotionally disturbed patients; hence they are more apt to see more emotionally disturbed patients. However, critics who are not familiar with such disturbances may miss the lesser disturbances and only recognize the major ones, since they are not as familiar with such problems. In any case, personality is more likely to be shaped by the patient's concepts and the family's attitudes and reactions to the seizures. Temporal lobe seizures often present with disturbances of memory, with hallucinations, and sometimes with what seems to be aggressive acting-out. The seizure may be followed by a stage of combative and destructive behavior during the recovery period when the patient is still confused. In his confusion the patient may misunderstand and misinterpret what is said and done. If the family, friends, and others around him do not recognize these as seizure-related symptoms, they may be unfair in their attitudes and reactions. Drugs also may bring out abnormal behaviors and emotions, especially those already present to a lesser degree before medication, but they may not be recognized as drug-related reactions. By adolescence, the patient, who is already burdened by the stresses of the seizures, now also experiences the normal adolescent crisis; he may not be able to cope with the combined stresses and his emotional stability may falter.

Tendencies The behavioral characteristics credited to the chronic temporal lobe epilepsy patient include any of the following symptoms: 1) intense but widely and rapidly changeable emotions, 2) slowed, repetitious, and rigid behaviors, 3) altered, usually depressed, sexual interests, or 4) tendencies toward developing psychiatric problems. However, the chronic temporal lobe epilepsy patient may also have an intact and relatively normal personality and behavior.

The temporal lobe seizure patient may show very strong and intense emotions. His emotional controls may be fragile. He may over-react and his responses may appear inappropriate. Basically, the patient may present with a good-natured, benign, and helpful personality, exhibiting a strong sense of ethics and justice. He may actively pursue moral, religious, or philosophical interests. Against this background may appear sudden explosive outbursts of anger, irritability, deep bouts of depression, or impulsive acting-out. These outbursts may be provoked by seemingly minor events.

Some patients present with a rigid and non-adaptable type of personality. The patient may be slowed in his responses to emotional stimuli, in his thinking, and in his efforts to adapt to new stimuli. His thinking, and also his speech, may be not only slow but also deliberate and excessive. He may continue to dwell on certain ideas, resisting change. Some patients dislike interruptions; they may have problems changing their thoughts. Some may become obsessed with a ritualistic orderliness, including a compulsive attention to detail. The patient may have problems distinguishing what is unimportant from what is important; he may dwell on trivia and overlook the significant. His behaviors may be performed over and over again, since he may have difficulties adapting to anything new or any different method of response. These problems are more common with seizure patients who have experienced brain damage, especially those whose problem began early in life. They may show up in the patient's speech and in his writing. He may be excessively wordy as he speaks or he may write lengthy diaries, notes, memoirs, or even books. In his overly detailed manner, he often overemphasizes the unimportant and glosses over the important.

Sexual interests and pursuits often are depressed in a temporal lobe seizure disorder. Rarely, the opposite extreme may occur. The level of sexual interests and arousal may normalize after temporal lobe surgery.

The temporal lobe seizure patient may be more prone to both minor and major psychiatric disturbances. There are various relationships between temporal lobe seizures and psychotic behaviors to be considered.

Many patients who have a temporal lobe seizure problem do not exhibit clear-cut signs of the various problems outlined. They may have overcome or suppressed the problem; they may have been able to cope with the stresses that otherwise might have produced the problem.

Growing Up The emotional over-reactions of the young child mellow as he grows to adulthood. The hyperactivity of early childhood may change into repetitive and persevering behavior by adolescence; sometimes the change is toward more delinquent behavior. Catastrophic rage reactions of childhood often become episodes of anger in adolescence. In the adult this tendency may mellow to mere irritability. Depression and suicidal tendencies become more common in later life.

Left and Right Temporal Lobe Syndromes The two brain halves differ in their style of thought processing. There may be significant differences in the related emotional behaviors. Each hemisphere may develop its own emotional reactions and behaviors, depending on that hemisphere's characteristic style of learning.

The left temporal lobe is usually involved in epilepsy more often than the right. Left temporal lobe seizures tend to appear at an earlier age than those on the right side. The left brain half is primarily in charge of processing language. A patient with a seizure disorder involving this left dominant hemisphere tends to be more introspective, reflective, and contemplative.

His behavior may be more verbally oriented. He may be less adept at detecting and interpreting emotional cues correctly. His misinterpretations may result in problems in interpersonal relationships as well as in the expression of his own feelings.

A left temporal lobe seizure patient may demonstrate ruminative intellectual tendencies. He may pursue religious or philosophical interests. He may become deeply concerned that external events influence his life and destiny. This can show up in his excessive note-taking and his overly detailed diaries.

The left temporal lobe patient may also tend to over-emphasize his faults, while minimizing his strengths and successes. He may over-report negative aspects of his behavior. Catastrophic reactions of anxiety and despair may appear when he is faced with a potential failure. The distorted relationships between the emotional centers and those thinking centers that depend on verbal language processes may cause the patient to be overly aware of his feelings, consequently exaggerating them to others. A left temporal lobe seizure patient may be more prone to develop a thought disturbance than a mood disturbance.

The psychiatric tendencies associated with the two kinds of temporal lobe seizure are outlined in Table 12.1.

The right hemisphere handles non-verbal thinking. A patient with a right temporal lobe seizure problem may have a more emotive disposition, which he displays outwardly. Such displays include anger, sadness, elation, euphoria, talkativeness about trivia, a rigid tendency toward repeating the same behaviors, and a strict adherence to rules. He may desire strict punishment for anyone who disobeys the rules. He may be more impulsive: his fragile emotions swing back and forth and are accompanied by acting-out behavior. This impulsivity often is directed outward in aggressive behavior or inward as depression.

The right temporal lobe seizure patient tends to minimize or deny proven socially unacceptable behaviors and documented aggressive acts. He tends to exaggerate his valued qualities. If he develops a psychiatric problem, it is more apt to be a mood disturbance than a thought disturbance.

Rage Reactions

A rage reaction is a sudden outburst of aggressive rage triggered by a seemingly minor frustration. It is seen in temporal lobe seizure problems of early onset and often following a brain insult or an excessively prolonged seizure. Rage reactions are not seizures. They may occur in people who do not have seizures and in whom normal EEGs are found. Rage reactions to minor frustrations may be due to a slowed and incomplete ability to cope with and adapt to stresses. A patient reacts without inhibition. His reaction is a prim-

Table 12.1. Psychiatric tendencies associated with temporal lobe seizures

Left Temporal Lobe	Right Temporal Lobe
SELF-DESCRIPTION	
Emphasizes faults	Exaggerates good qualities
Minimizes strengths	Denies disapproved behaviors
Tarnishes his image	Tries to build a good image
ORIENTATION	
Introspective and contemplative	Gregarious and impulsive
Intellectual ruminations	Externalized emotions
Religious pursuits	Anger
Philosophical interests	Sadness
Sense of personal destiny	Euphoria and elation
Feels events influence life and destiny	Talkative about details
	Repetitious
REACTIONS	
Verbal expression of ideas	Non-verbal reactions
Excessively detailed speech and language	Emotional with wide swings
	Aggressive (often denied)
EMOTIONAL PROBLEMS	
Thought disturbances	Mood disturbances
Catastrophic fears and despairs	
Paranoid schizophrenia	Manic depressive
Hyperactivity	Impulsive, aggressive

itive, immature response rather than a more mature effort to adapt. The patient may appear docile and submissive between the attacks, providing that he has no other behavior problems. After an attack he may seem contrite, ashamed, forgetful, and confused. He may even deny the attack.

The problem of rage reactions may relate to brain damage involving the temporal and adjacent underneath portions of the frontal lobe as well as more central portions relating to emotions. The rages do not respond to anticonvulsant medications. They may be partially suppressed by tranquilizers, but these drugs in turn may aggravate the seizures, slow down learning, and inhibit the development of needed coping skills. Behavior modification is the desired therapy. The rages of childhood tend to mature to mere episodes of irritability by adulthood.

Psychoses and Seizures

Major behavior disturbances and psychomotor seizure symptoms may seem superficially similar. Psychotic hallucinations are often threatening, consisting of voices making negative comments about the seizures, whereas the seizure hallucinations are less threatening; the patient with seizure hallucinations realizes that they are not real. Emotional outbursts, peculiar sensations, and bizarre thoughts can be seen with either problem, but with seizures the episodes are much briefer.

Types Psychotic behavior can develop in an epileptic patient at any time. Some psychotic states appear with an accompanying disturbance of consciousness, whereas others appear when the patient is relatively alert and conscious. When the patient presents in a confused, non-alert psychotic state, the behavior may be caused by ongoing absence staring episodes or psychomotor seizures, by drug reactions, or by brain damage itself. A brief psychotic state may be part of the recovery-confusional state following a seizure. The patient is more apt to be delerious in a temporal lobe seizure status, with drug reactions, or in a post-ictal state; by comparison, the patient in an absence state of continuous staring seizures is more apt to appear to be in a confused stupor than in an agitated delerium.

Some seizure patients present with an alert but psychotic behavior. The psychosis may be brief, but it may recur in further episodes. Such episodes may precede the seizure, appear with it, or recur at periods unrelated to the occurrence of a seizure. The patient may present with an agitated, hyperactive, manic state or a discouraged, depressed state. Sometimes the psychotic episodes and seizure episodes may alternate. More prolonged and chronic psychotic states, occasionally with episodic increases, may also be seen. These include paranoid syndromes, schizophrenic-like syndromes, manic-depressive psychoses, and psychoses characterized by a mental and emotional regression to a more immature level of functioning. In psychiatric reviews, left temporal lobe seizures may be more associated with a paranoid schizophrenic psychosis and right temporal lobe seizures with a manic depressive problem.

Causes The exact relationship between a seizure and a psychosis is unclear. The problems may occur together by chance. The epilepsy or the drugs used in managing the seizures may trigger an inherited tendency toward psychosis. The seizure and the psychosis may both be symptoms of an underlying brain lesion. The psychotic state may be the manifestation of an unrecognized seizure or it may be an emotional reaction to the seizure disorder and its related problems. The psychosis can be due to a drug reaction or the drugs used for the psychosis may activate a seizure problem.

TREATMENT OF EMOTIONAL DISTURBANCES

The goals of therapy in seizure patients who present with significant emotional or behavioral disturbances are to control the overt seizures and to improve the behaviors. The anticonvulsant drug itself may bring about improvement, although it may also have no effect or it may even make the behavior worse, with the appearance of moodiness, irritability, or agitation. There are three types of therapeutic approaches: 1) drugs, 2) psychotherapy, and 3) surgery.

In the hyperkinetic syndrome, the main therapy must include behavioral counseling and modification, no matter what the cause of the syndrome. With true hyperactivity, stimulants may be helpful. However, if drugs are used without the behavioral counseling, the long-range outcome may be poor. Tranquilizers may be ineffective and may trigger seizures, as can the stimulants. If they are used until effective behavioral therapy can be established, Mellaril, Valium, or Librium may be the most helpful.

As with other neurologic problems, emotional stress, anxiety, tension, or agitation may increase the seizures. Anxiety-relieving methods, such as relaxation techniques, crisis intervention, counseling, or use of Valium may be useful, both for the crisis and for improving consequent seizure control. Behavioral counseling should be ongoing in order to help the patient learn to cope with his problems. More vigorous psychologic management of temporal lobe epilepsy problems, including behavior modification techniques, is becoming a valuable help in a rounded seizure management approach.

Irritability may respond to Tegretol, although a major tranquilizer or anti-anxiety drug may be needed with severe cases. Patients with marked swings in mood between depression and elation also may respond to Tegretol. This drug is especially helpful with depressed states.

A psychosis due to a seizure status responds best to an appropriate increase in the anticonvulsant medications. If the psychotic state is due to a drug reaction, discontinuing the aggravating drug should stop the psychosis. If the psychosis appears when the seizures become controlled, a cautious reduction of the anticonvulsant may cause the psychotic behavior to disappear as a few seizures reappear. If the anticonvulsant is increased rather than decreased, the psychotic state in these alternating attacks is not helped and may be made worse. With this so-called alternating psychosis (alternating with seizures), the EEG is the most normal when the psychosis is the most active. This phenomenon is not common with chronic psychoses. Psychotherapy is the desired treatment for epileptic psychoses, especially the chronic ones. Tegretol may aggravate the alternating psychoses but often it is helpful with other psychotic reactions, especially when used in combination with antipsychotic medication. These antipsychotic medications, such as the major tranquilizers, if used alone, may trigger the seizures. It may be that the benefit of the tranquilizer in an alternating psychosis is to activate the seizure enough to allow the psychosis to disappear. It is best to use an anticonvulsant along with the antipsychotic medication. A balanced combination of the anticonvulsant and the antipsychotic drug along with active psychotherapy is the desired management, especially for episodic psychoses. The antipsychotic drugs, especially those associated with reduced consciousness, appear to reduce restlessness. Paranoid symptoms may improve but seldom completely disappear.

Although not used primarily for the control of emotional and behavioral problems, temporal lobectomy can have many beneficial effects on such problems. Not only is the seizure control often improved, but aggressive traits are often reduced and depressed sexuality tends to normalize. There is little change in the religious and philosophical drives, the repetitive behaviors, and perseverative deliberate thinking trends, or in the psychoses themselves.

Considerations

Whether the emotional disturbance or behavioral problem is the result of the epilepsy, the underlying brain lesion, the drug, or the environmental attitudes and influences, the patient with such a problem needs help. There are certain obvious facts. There is a significant increase in emotional and behavioral problems in the epileptic patient. The environment plays an active role in the development of the personality of the seizure patient but it is probably not the only factor. Emotional and behavioral problems can become more handicapping than the seizure problem. The patient with such problems needs help, no matter what the cause may be. Proper therapy of a seizure patient extends beyond just controlling the seizures, it consists also of behavioral intervention. Early intervention and counseling guidance, born of awareness of potential needs of the patient, may help by lessening the environmental stresses on the developing personality.

THE HOME

The family of the seizure patient is often overwhelmed by a diagnosis of epilepsy. The parents want to know why their child is epileptic, although the mother often suspects that she may be somehow responsible, having given birth to the child. The mother is likely to alternate between being dismayed, feeling incapable of caring for an epileptic child, and reacting with calm, help-seeking acceptance. She may accept the problem as the will of fate. Most of the family's knowledge about seizures appears to come from medical personnel. This source is felt to be satisfactory. The mother often feels the seizures are due to a birth injury, although she may consider an illness during pregnancy or early life or a trauma or an illness suffered by the child as other possible causes. The mother tends to pursue other sources of information. She relies on her own observations especially, but she also learns by reading or talking about the problems of epilepsy with her husband, her relatives, or her friends.

The home attitudes affect the child's self-concept and self-image. Often the parents are filled with misunderstandings. Middle-class families may be worried about the impact on the family activities. Lower-class parents may worry about their ability to provide proper care for the patient.

Some parents resent the stigma, the inconvenience, the cost, and the restrictins caused by the epilepsy. More often the parents feel insecure and uncertain about what is normal and what is abnormal, what to do and what not to do. They may be overly sensitive to minor deviations from normal, yet overlook or deny major disturbances. The parents may appear hostile and demanding as a cover for their anxiety. Overlooking the hostile cover and reassuring them about their fears may reveal that they are worried parents, seeking help, and not a nuisance.

Parents feel an epileptic child requires more attention. The parents develop increased concerns over what should and shouldn't be done. The seizure patient seems to develop more behavioral problems than the other children in the family. The immediate concerns are over the safety of the child, the fear of triggering a life-threatening seizure if the child is disciplined or of provoking an attack if the child does not get his demands. The parents also worry about how to handle a major seizure attack. Long-range concerns include problems of learning and earning and of the child getting along with others. Specific problems anticipated by the parents include watching for seizures day and night, explaining the epilepsy to teachers and to others who come in contact with the patient, dealing with public opinion, avoiding activities that might cause a seizure, and protecting the child from real or imagined harm. To handle all this takes time and energy. Consequently the rest of the family tends to be neglected while the patient is over-protected. Occasionally a patient is rejected by his family rather than over-protected.

Over-Management, Over-Protection, Over-Indulgence, Over-Restriction

The parents' relationship to the child is most important. Parents of a handicapped child are often insecure about their handling of the child. They fear that they may do more harm than good. This is often felt more with a lesser handicap than with a major one. A major fear is that anything that causes anger, frustration, or any emotional upset may trigger a seizure. Consequently, the parent tends to avoid anything that might possibly trigger the seizure. The child may sense this and manipulate it to his own advantage. He can become capricious, demanding, and self-centered. He learns to get but never to give. He grows up believing that society will provide for his desires just as his parents have... and he is shocked when this does not happen. Over-indulgent parents are often manipulated by the child. The child may refuse to eat, refuse to go to bed, demand to sleep with a favored parent, refuse medicines or tests, throw temper tantrums, or even fake seizures in order to obtain his desires.

Over-indulgent parents of a child with epilepsy may be suffering from both anger and guilt. They suspect that they may be responsible for their child's problem. This suspicion may lead to a near obsessional desire to protect the child from any further harm. The parents may keep the child under constant surveillance, day and night. To keep the child from harm they may impose excessive and unrealistic restrictions that the child must either surrender to or rebel against. Medical and school personnel may unwittingly support these efforts. The child often finds himself not accepted by others due to his parents' over-protection and his own distorted behavior. This leads to a poor development of social relationships, resulting in an isolated, immature individual.

By adulthood the over-indulged and over-protected patient has difficulties coping with daily life. He may not have developed the emotional maturity and motivation needed to hold a job despite good seizure control. Early intervention, including intensive counseling and guidance from the very beginning, when the diagnosis is first suspected, is necessary to avoid this. Often the parents initially resist expressing their difficulties managing the problems of refusal to obey, of hyperactivity, and of temper outbursts. If the parents can be helped to recognize their own feelings and frustrations, they then can begin to deal with them, trying alternate approaches. Although individual ongoing counseling with each family is important, sometimes drawing a group of parents and other family members together in a group session may help to open up hesitant family members as various members of the group begin to share both frustrations and ideas. Individuals in such a group can build support for each other.

The Vulnerable Child Syndrome A child who is handicapped, who at some time has undergone a life-threatening insult, or who reminds the parents of another family member who was handicapped or has died may be seen by the parent as unrealistically fragile and vulnerable to harm. Epilepsy in childhood is a major trigger of this vulnerability, particularly if the parent has both good and bad feelings toward the child. This often creates further fears of possible harm to the child. The parent and child may have difficulties in separating without undue anxiety, especially when the child goes to school or is hospitalized. Such a child often acts immature, since the parents treat him like a younger child for fear that he might grow up and die. The child tends to have difficulties in school and often is an underachiever. The family appears overly concerned with trivial health matters. There is a strong tendency to spoil the child. Little evidence of disciplinary efforts is seen. The parents' reactions to the child may include shock, denial, cure searching, guilt, over-protection, and resentment of the behavioral problems without any effort to control them. The home life ends up being very disturbed. The mother practices "smother love" rather than mother love.

This problem must be recognized. The family must be convinced that the child is not as ill as they envision. They must recognize and deal with the real problem through counseling. Imagined worries must be dispelled, confidence built up, and realistic management encouraged. It is far better to prevent this syndrome from developing by giving proper explanation and support and having help available from the very beginning, when the diagnosis is first suspected.

The Household

The mother, in her guilt reaction, may dedicate her life to "making it up" to the child. She finds this life to be confining and restrictive. Often she ends the prolonged day exhausted. She may seek support from a neighbor or friend or she may follow religious or philosophical pursuits to gain understanding of why this has happened. Occasionally she will turn to the medical services, schools, or parent groups for help. If she can obtain the needed support, she often responds in a positive manner, especially if she senses a positive interest that might be of help to her child.

There is a tendency for the family triad of father, mother, and epileptic child to break down to a "two plus one" (mother and child, plus the father) relationship. The father may voluntarily exclude himself or he may subconsciously be excluded by the mother. A father may become more responsive, helpful, and supporting, or he may reject the child in shame and denial of any problem. Sometimes a father will place the blame on the mother. Occasionally the diagnosis of epilepsy will lead to a divorce — a definite rearrangement to a "two plus one" relationship. Some fathers refuse to help with care because they are jealous of the attention that the child receives. Others may participate actively in the attention and spoiling. It is always desirable to have the father present at each medical examination and especially in counseling.

There appears to be a greater disruption in the home environment of epileptic children with significant emotional disturbances, but the problems of epilepsy may also promote family closeness and discussion. There tends to be more agreement about the upbringing and management of the epileptic child, despite the father's tendency to adopt a negative attitude.

Family activities are quite altered. Outings tend to be restricted, especially if they risk the embarrassment of a seizure. Since they may not entrust their child to a babysitter, the family tends to stay home, and often family members feel tied down.

The child's brothers and sisters often appear to be understanding and helpful, although they may be jealous of the extra attention he receives. Sometimes the siblings are teased about their epileptic brother or sister. The mother's tendency to neglect other family members in favor of care of the patient may increase jealousies. Frequently the siblings are given extra chores and responsibilities, whereas the epileptic child is given fewer duties.

Medical Help The parents turn to the medical staff for help. They may not receive the assistance or counseling they seek. The parents complain that they receive quick, superficial, short, or vague explanations, filled with difficult medical terms, from a physician who seems uninterested. The family is left with no chance to ask questions. The doctor seems to be unavailable when he is needed. The parents end up with varying and confusing opinions and diagnoses. Sometimes they are falsely reassured that the child will grow out of the problem. When not satisfied, the family may go to another physician or may embark on a search among physicians for the desired help.

One problem in seizure control is cooperation in the regular administration of the medicines prescribed. Some parents who feel insecure in their own abilities may over-react in a dogmatic fashion. They tend to feel that they, not the physician, know what is best in the management of the medicines. Thus they alter the drugs on their own, rather than following the prescribed directions. A simple, careful explanation, including the goals and rationale for the prescribed method, accompanied by ample time to discuss questions and establish a good follow-up, is needed to overcome this problem.

Counseling Many families desire active counseling. A majority of these families can obtain it. The major concerns for which counseling is sought usually are about behavioral management. Occasionally genetic counseling regarding any future children is desired.

Management Problems, abnormal attitudes, and distorted reactions are much more evidenced in children with uncontrolled seizures. Medical personnel can be more effective if they are sensitive to the concerns and questions of the patient and the family. The physician or another medical team member should take time to give full, simple explanations and assurances as they are needed and desired. Interest, concern, and availability should be evidenced by the staff. They just either handle directly or refer for appropriate services any problems that appear in the seizure patient. Referrals may be for psychological help, for counseling, or for the handling of any other problems that may arise.

The parents' insecurity often is coupled with guilt, resentment, and rejection. Ideally the parent(s) should be involved in the care of the patient during the initial seizure hospitalization. Otherwise they tend to feel that they have failed their child and that the medical staff has taken over to give better care until the problem has receded to the level that the parents are capable of handling. Involving the parents as part of the care team helps preserve their self-concepts. During the initial evaluation, counseling sessions to promote understanding may prevent future problems as well as establish better management. The staff must always work with the patient actively and not just with the family.

Counseling should begin with noting the family's attitudes toward discipline and responsibility, looking for signs of indulgence, over-protection, or over-restriction, as well as any hints of rejection. The families should be encouraged to express their feelings and frustrations. The counselor needs to provide information about epilepsy, about methods in management of all of the needs of the epileptic child, including guidance toward better emotional maturation and encouragement toward the development of confidence and independence. The family may need to be referred for further help in family planning. They may need guidance in the management of the child as well as in handling the impact of the epilepsy on the family.

INSTITUTIONALIZATION

An epileptic patient may be placed in an institution if he has other severe handicaps, if the family cannot cope or manage him at home, or if training and management services that are not available at home are available through the institution. The placement may be permanent or it may be a temporary training period aimed at developing enough basic skills and improved functioning so that the patient can be handled at home and may be able to enter into local programs.

Institutionalization creates conflicting emotions in the family. They feel guilty for failing the patient and having to place him elsewhere. They also feel relieved of the epileptic stigma and burden. They hope that the experts in the institution will be able to improve seizure control and overall functioning. This hope reassures them about their decision to institutionalize the patient.

Yet the patient may not improve, at least not to the expectations of the family. Relieved of the constant reminder of the daily care, the family begins to reconsider. They see that the seizures and related problems continue without the hoped-for improvement. They begin to lose confidence in the institution. They begin to build up the once-shattered confidence in their own efforts in the past as they begin to criticize the institution's efforts. Doubt regarding the decision to institutionalize begins to appear.

As the family's confidence in the institution drops, the family begins to find flaws and faults. They may seek reassurance and support to justify their criticisms. They may support their own rationalizations to the point that they decide to reclaim their child from the institution. The cycle of "I cannot do as well as they can!" "I did just as well as they did!" "I can do better than they can!" begins again.

The institution should understand the ambivalent feelings of the family. The institutional personnel should offer full explanations, outline goals, methods, and expectations, and give periodic progress reports to the family. The personnel in the institutions must be sensitive and responsive to the questions and concerns of the family. Involving the family in care whenever possible may be useful.

The institution should develop an individualized rehabilitative program for the patient. The family should be involved in the plan. If deinstitutionalization is a potential option, the family must be prepared and trained to re-assume the management role. The overall goal should be better function. The parents should be aware of this at all times; their awareness may be reinforced by frequently reporting to them the progress being made.

Efforts also should be made to upgrade institutional management, but pressures for improvement must be accompanied by a means of financing this. Many institutions are asked to perform miracles with minimum financial support. Whenever possible, the institution should contract for assistance from nearby major medical clinics and other consultative services. An available information and referral source for more complex or acute major problems should be established. Affiliations with medical schools can promote better care as well as ongoing in-service training, upgrading the care and understanding of the institutional personnel. The experience of working with an institution often proves rewarding to medical school personnel.

Smaller institutions may not be able to provide basic seizure control services, including EEGs and anticonvulsant blood level measurements. However, these may be contracted for with a medical center. As an alternative, several institutions may share these services. Such efforts have been shown to reduce seizures significantly, to reduce deaths among the institutionalized epileptics, to reduce costs, to improve functioning of the patients, and to promote successful discharge of more patients from the institution.

At the time of the discharge, appropriate plans must be made to see that the medical care, as well as the social and rehabilitative programs, are continued at home. The gains of the institution should not be lost just because a continuation of the care was not established when the patient returned home. Again, the family must be included as an important part of the management program, both in the preparation for and then after the actual discharge. Follow-up checks may be indicated to see that the patient is still receiving the needed services after he has left the institution. Some institutions may consider brief out-patient review sessions for the family and as a check up on patients, to ensure that the progress is being maintained and to help support the family.

ENVIRONMENT

The epileptic child's experience outside the home tends to be one of rejection. The growing child meets this in his neighborhood, at school, in his town, and later on, in the work environment (see Chapter 14). The main causes of the rejection are ignorance about epilepsy, fear that a seizure will occur in the presence of the fearful onlooker, and prejudices about what has been heard but not really known about seizures. This attitude may cause further emotional stresses.

The Neighborhood

The epileptic child may not be accepted by the other children in the neighborhood, especially if the seizures are not well controlled. The child may have more difficulties in getting along with others. His undesirable behaviors may cause him to be excluded from group activities and to be rejected.

The School

The school may seek to exclude the child from attending class by providing at-home private teaching and by encouraging its use as a desirable alternative. The reasons given for not having the child in school are many, but they most often center on the epilepsy or the behavioral problems. Even the physician may approve of this arrangement. However, this approach is often undesirable: not only may the amount and quality of tutoring be inferior, but also the child loses out on opportunities for social interactions, which he especially needs.

The school administration has fears about its liability for any trauma suffered on the school grounds. Administrators fear the stigma of the epilepsy and the class disruption an attack may cause. Consequently, even if the school is unable to exclude the child, the personnel may unconsciously aggravate the child's emotional problems through their unspoken rejection. The personnel may not cooperate in allowing midday medications to be given. This attitude may cause the child to become reluctant to take his medications in public, especially after a school official has created a fuss about the medicine. The physician could help avoid this by either altering the dosage schedule to avoid midday medicines or else working with the school personnel to overcome their reluctance. It is obviously better if they can adopt a calm, understanding, helpful attitude.

The Teacher Although the teacher may be uncomfortable about epilepsy, she usually does not blame the child for it, realizing that the child cannot help having this disability. She may be equally as disturbed by the child's behavior, but, unless it is severe, she tends to tolerate it, believing it to be another symptom of the seizures. One item that teachers heap blame upon is the medications. Any learning failures, any undesirable behaviors, and any peculiar emotional outbursts are blamed on the medications. Helping the teacher to learn about epilepsy and about the child's medications, and involving her as part of the team, may reduce her concerns. The teacher who is knowledgeable about epilepsy can be a valuable aid in monitoring for any genuine drug side effects, behavior problems, or other possible difficulties requiring attention. If she functions as a member of the care team, she may take more interest and thus be more helpful to the child.

The Parents' View of the School   In their over-protectiveness, the parents fear that the child might experience physical or emotional harm at school. They feel that the personnel are not able to manage the problems of epilepsy, including special educational needs. They fear that stresses and possible ridicule at school will aggravate the seizures and the behavioral problems. They sense that their child is neither understood nor wanted. They fear that the school will not cooperate in good care for the child, including the giving of the medicines. They feel that their child would be safer at home.

The child seems to have fewer problems in school and to be better accepted if the seizure problem is well accepted at home and if his family requires that he be active and productive. School behavior problems relate to home behavioral management. Parents are most satisfied with the school and their child's educational placement if the seizures are controlled, if the child has no learning problems, and especially if the personnel seem interested and anxious to help with the child's problems.

Parents often feel and expect that the school personnel know more about epilepsy and its consequences than they really do. Efforts need to be made to increase the training of the school staff regarding epilepsy and its consequences.

The Child's View of the School   After the home experience of over-protection, over-indulgence, and under-expectation, the child may fear going to school, where he anticipates he will be expected to perform well and to behave. At school the child tends to become more anxious and vulnerable to various stresses. His attention may be spread thin; he becomes distractable. Boys especially seem to isolate themselves. The child may also sense the attitudes, fears, and rejection of his classmates. He may become depressed. He feels safer and more secure at home, where he can have his own way. This may be especially true if some of his classmates ridicule his attacks. The child may manipulate the fears of his parents and of the school in order to be allowed to stay in the safer home.

The Classmates   His classmates may fear the seizures but they often do not tease or ridicule the epileptic child. They tend to exclude him and reject him, but more often because of his behavior than because of his epilepsy. However, the child who is more self-conscious and on guard because of his epilepsy may misinterpret what others do and say as being ridicule. The parents of the classmates also may fear psychological harm to their own children should they see a seizure.

Ideal Management   Teachers and other school personnel should be given the basic knowledge of epilepsy and its associated problems as part of their basic training. They should be given resources for further learning. The patient's physician should work with and help the teacher. The ideal medical team would include an educator liaison to promote cooperation with the school authorities in patient care. The school staff should show interest, concern, and helpfulness toward both the child and his worried parents. All ridicule and rejection should be avoided. Cooperative management includes helping with medications. Such an approach often gains the parents' confidence. Should a seizure occur in a classroom, the teacher has an opportunity to teach by example the correct attitudes toward and handling of a handicap.

A child should be put in the type of class best meeting his educational and social needs. The physician and teacher should work together, monitoring for possible seizures, drug reactions, or other problems, Behavior problems should not be tolerated. Such problems must be modified if the child is to learn to succeed in later life. Modifying these behaviors should be done by the medical team, the school team, and the parents. A successful school experience develops when the parents and the school personnel are both convinced that each is concerned, competent, encouraging, supportive, and working to help the child.

CONCLUSION

Multiple factors, including disturbed brain functions related to the seizure, the drugs, or underlying brain problems, as well as the attitudes toward and management of the seizure patient by others about him tend to result in disturbed emotions in a majority of seizure patients. Often these attitudes lead to disturbed behaviors that can become more handicapping than the seizure problem. The problems may be minor and easily solved through counseling and guidance, or they may be major, requiring intensive behavioral intervention. Good seizure care includes active work with such problems in addition to attempts to control the seizures.

REFERENCES AND SUGGESTED READINGS

General

Aird, R. B., and D. M. Woodbury. 1974. The Management of Epilepsy, Chapter 6, pp. 304-358. Charles C Thomas, Springfield, Ill.

(The) Commission for the Control of Epilepsy and Its Consequences, 1975-77. The Plans for Action on Epilepsy, Vol. 1. DHEW Publication No. (NIS 78-276). U.S. Department of Health, Education, and Welfare, National Institutes of Health, Office of Scientific and Health Reports, NINCDS-NIH, Bethesda, Md. 20014.

Gomez, M. R., and D. W. Klass. 1972. Seizures and other paroxysmal disorders in infants and children. Current Problems in Pediatrics, Vol. 2. Year Book Medical Publishers, Inc., Chicago.

Sands, H., and F. C. Minters. 1977. The Epilepsy Fact Book. F. A. Davis Co., Philadelphia. 116 pp.
Solomon, G. E., and F. Plum. 1976. Clinical Management of Seizures, Chapter 7. W. B. Saunders Company, Philadelphia.
Stores, G. 1975. Behavioral effects of anti-epileptic drugs. Dev. Med. Child. Neurol. 17:647-658.
Wright, G. N. 1975. Epilepsy Rehabilitation. Little, Brown & Company, Boston. 275 pp.

Childhood Problems

Hartlage, L. C., J. B. Green, and L. Offut. 1972. Dependency in epileptic children. Epilepsia 13:27-30.
Svoboda, W. B. 1975. The hyperkinetic syndrome. W. Va. Med. J. 71:347-351.

Environment

Baley, C. 1972. Social prejudices and the adjustment of people with epilepsy. Epilepsia 13:33-45.
Boshes, L. D., and H. W. Kienst. 1972. Community aspects of epilepsy — a modern reappraisal. Epilepsia 13:31-32.
Caveness, W. F., H. H. Merritt, and G. H. Gallup, Jr. 1974. A survey of public attitudes toward epilepsy in 1974 with an indication of trends over the past twenty-five years. Epilepsia 15:523-536.

Family

Clausen, J. 1977. Psychological intervention with parents of children with epilepsy. In: J. K. Penry (ed.), Epilepsy, the Eighth International Symposium, pp. 215-238. Raven Press, New York.
Green, J., and A. J. Solnit. 1964. Reaction to the threatened loss of a child: A vulnerable child syndrome. Pediatrics 34:58-66.
Lerman, P. 1977. The concept of preventive rehabilitation in childhood epilepsy: A plea against overprotection and overindulgence. In: J. K. Penry (ed.), Epilepsy, the Eighth International Symposium, pp. 265-268. Raven Press, New York.
Nhan, N. 1975. The epileptic child and his family (report). National Children's Rehabilitation Center, Leesburg, Virginia. 97 pp.

Individuals

Lennox, W. G. 1960. Epilepsy and Related Disorders, Chapter 20, pp. 659-699. Little, Brown & Company, Boston.
Singer, H. S., and J. M. Freeman. 1975. Seizures in adolescents. Med. Clin. North Am. 59:1461-1472.

Institutional

Freeman, J. M. 1977. Approaches to Improved Care of Institutionalized Epileptic Persons. The Developmental Disabilities Training and Technical Assistance Center, University of Maryland, Baltimore. 30 pp.

Medical

Lennox, W. G. 1960. Epilepsy and Related Disorders, Chapter 24, pp. 785-797. Little, Brown & Company, Boston.

Psychiatric Problems, Major and Minor

Bech, P., K. K. Pedersen, N. Simonsen, and M. Lund. 1977. Personality traits in epilepsy. In: J. K. Penry (ed.), Epilepsy, The Eighth International Symposium, pp. 257-263. Raven Press, New York.

Blumer, D. 1972. Neuropsychiatric aspects of psychomotor and other forms of epilepsy in childhood. In: S. Livingston (ed.), Comprehensive Management of Epilepsy in Infancy, Childhood and Adolescence, Chapter 12, pp. 486-497. Charles C Thomas, Springfield, Ill.

Blumer, D., and K. Levin. 1977. Psychiatric Complications in the Epilepsies: Current Research and Treatment. Proceedings of the Conference on Psychiatric Disorders in Epilepsy, No. 15, 1976. McLean Hospital Journal, Special Issue — 1977. McLean Hospital, Belmont, Mass., and Geigy Pharmaceuticals, Division of CIBA-Geigy Corporation, Ardsley, New York. 103 pp.

Bruens, J. W. 1974. Psychoses in epilepsy. In: O. Magnus and A. M. Lorentz de Haas (eds.), The Epilepsies, Chapter 32, pp. 593-610. P. J. Vincken and G. W. Bruyn (eds.), Handbook of Clinical Neurology, Vol. 15. Elsevier-North Holland Publishing Company, New York.

Flor-Henry, P. 1972. Ictal and interictal psychiatric manifestations in epilepsy: Specific or non-specific. Epilepsia 13:773-783.

Milner, B. 1975. Psychological aspects of focal epilepsy and its neurosurgical management. In: D. P. Purpura, J. K. Penry, and R. D. Walter (eds.), Advances in Neurology, Vol. 8, Chapter 15, pp. 299-321. Raven Press, New York.

Ponds, D. A. 1974. Epilepsy and personality disorders. In: B. Magnus and A. M. Lorentz de Haas (eds.), The Epilepsies, Chapter 32, pp. 593-610. P. J. Vincken and G. W. Bruyn (eds.), Handbook of Clinical Neurology, Vol. 15. Elsevier-North Holland Publishing Company, New York.

Taylor, D. C. 1977. Epilepsia and the sinister side of schizophrenia. Dev. Med. Child Neurol. 19:403-406.

School

Hackney, A., and D. C. Taylor. 1976. A teacher's questionnaire description of epileptic children. Epilepsia 17:275-282.

Hartlage, L. C., and J. B. Green. 1972. The relationship of parental attitudes to academic and social achievement in epileptic children. Epilepsia 13:21-26.

Lennox, W. G. 1960. Epilepsia and Related Disorders, Chapter 27, pp. 919-999. Little, Brown & Company, Boston.

Pazzaglia, P., and L. Frank-Pazzaglia. 1976. Record in grade school of pupils with epilepsy: An epidemiological study. Epilepsia 17:361-366.

Stores, G. 1977. Behavior disturbances and types of epilepsy in children attending ordinary school. In: J. K. Penry (ed.), Epilepsy, the Eighth International Symposium, pp. 245-249. Raven Press, New York.

Temporal Lobe Seizures

Bear, D. M., and P. Fedio. 1977. Quantitative analysis of interictal behavior in temporal lobe epilepsy. Arch. Neurol. 34:454-467.

McIntyre, M., P. B. Pritchard III, and C. T. Lombroso. 1976. Left and right temporal lobe epileptics: A controlled investigation of some psychological differences. Epilepsia 17:377-386.

Ounsted, C., J. Lindsay, and R. Norman. 1966. Biologic Factors in Temporal Lobe Epilepsy. Clinics in Developmental Medicine, No. 22. William Heinemann Medical Books Ltd., London. 135 pp.

Rodin, E. A., M. Katz, and K. Lennox. 1976. Differences between patients with temporal lobe seizures and those with other forms of seizure attacks. Epilepsia 17:313-320.

13
EPILEPSY AND LEARNING PROBLEMS

The main handicaps of epilepsy are not the seizures; they are the learning and later earning problems and the social and behavioral difficulties. Learning problems and behavioral disturbances are both present in roughly half of the epileptic individuals. A similar percentage of children have difficulties in making a normal adjustment to school. A significant number of epileptic children do not achieve up to expectations and their potential in school. Children with learning or behavioral complications of their epilepsy are at special risk for problems in school. Even when a cause of the seizure disorder is not known, the epileptic patient often shows some evidence of a learning deficit. If the cause of the epilepsy is known, this tendency is significantly greater, especially if there is known brain damage.

School problems in part may be due to the negative attitudes of the teacher and the classmates. They see the child as different. Obvious seizures usually are not missed. Minor attacks, such as staring spells, may be overlooked or even occasionally frankly denied by a teacher or parent. Rarely, a teacher may resist the diagnosis of a seizure if she feels she cannot handle an epileptic pupil in her classroom.

Learning problems may be due to unrecognized and subtle learning disabilities, which appear to be fairly common in the seizure patient. Learning difficulties also may be due to a depressed or deteriorating intelligence, to a drug reaction or intoxication, to behavioral and emotional disturbances, to unrecognized seizure activity, or to improper teaching attitudes and methods relative to the child's needs. Often the cause proves to be a mixture of factors.

Children with seizures of early onset are more likely to develop significant learning problems. The epilepsy may somehow interfere with intellectual development. The effects of a long-term seizure problem, its emotional stigma, and chronic usage of the anticonvulsant drugs also may be factors. Overt brain damage in early life has a more impairing effect than do comparable damaging influences occurring later in life. This is especially true if the patient develops epilepsy as another symptom of the damage. Both the basic thought processes and the problem-solving abilities appear to be affected. The patient may have difficulties adapting to new situations and challenges.

Major motor seizures may be associated with a greater impairment in psychologic functions than are focal, psychomotor, or absence attacks. However, psychomotor seizures often prove more handicapping, since they tend to produce distortions and blocks to the learning processes, with consequent effects on the related emotional and behavioral development. There appear to be the fewest problems with learning with simple focal and absence seizures. A unilateral seizure problem can be as handicapping as a psychomotor attack.

Undetected and untreated learning problems often result in non-learning or underachievement; they can cause later problems in employment and in social adjustment. Early detection and successful remediation may avoid such consequences. Improved overall seizure management has been shown to result in a drastic reduction of school problems.

BEHAVIORAL INTERFERENCES WITH LEARNING (see also Chapter 12)

Teachers describe many epileptic children as inattentive, distractable, restless, constantly fidgeting, or having poor concentration. This may be due to a behavioral problem, unrecognized seizures, a disturbed learning process, or a drug reaction. Yet behavior problems are not a common cause of learning difficulties; they are more apt to be the consequences of frustrations due to non-learning. Unrecognized seizures and drug reactions are infrequent causes of these problems.

Hyperactivity is often ascribed to the epileptic child, usually because of his difficulties with learning. The child becomes anxious and discouraged. He may be distracted by something more interesting. He may be looking for an escape from the difficult learning problem. He may be confused by the task and look around for answers elsewhere. He may be on guard for any threatening stimuli, manifesting a great deal of anxiety. The extra effort needed to overcome some difficult tasks may be stressful to him. He may become increasingly anxious and fidgety if he feels trapped in a situation with which he cannot cope. All these activities are usually superficially labeled as hyperactivity. Yet, careful attention to the quality of the attention as well as the quantity of the inattention may show that the child is attending, but not to the tasks; he is avoiding the task, watching something he is worried about, looking for an escape, searching for help, or he is plainly anxious. The stresses of this learning frustration and behavior may increase the number of seizures.

Other problems include poor memory recall. The child may also have difficulty with solving problems. His work approaches often are disorganized. He does not get his work done in the assigned time. Such behaviors suggest possible learning disabilities in need of help. Epileptic children with such problems often derive great profit from special educational help in organizing work habits, overcoming learning blocks, and applying the newly gained skills to tasks. Often behavioral modification techniques may be useful as a part of this approach.

UNRECOGNIZED SEIZURES

Unrecognized generalized seizure disorders may interfere with attention and learning if the bursts are very frequent or significantly prolonged. The presence of a significantly abnormal EEG with abnormal bursts may be associated with a greater degree of learning difficulties, even if no seizure activity is apparent. The type of discharge may correlate more with the type as well as the risks for a specific learning problem than it does with any specific behavioral problem. The school teacher may see a child staring in the class. If the child is underachieving, she may suspect a possible seizure problem and refer him for an evaluation. Staring episodes lasting more than a few minutes are probably not epileptic. Absence seizures usually last less than a minute or two. Unless the absence attacks are very frequent, such as hundreds of times a day, they usually do not significantly interfere with learning. There is no correlation of absence seizures with reading skills. Missing school because of seizures and medical appointments, or because of other health problems, such as behavioral disturbance, does not correlate with depressed reading achievements.

A major question is whether overt seizures are the only ongoing disturbance of brain function. Seizure bursts on the EEG may not be large enough or last long enough to produce any seizure symptoms. This discharge, if located in a vital brain center that is involved in processing learning, may interfere with the child's learning. It has been estimated that, for every seizure seen, there may be at least 50 or more brief bursts or discharges, some lasting only a fraction of a second. These may be important as far as learning is concerned. There have been cases reported in which a patient was not doing well in school and was found to have an EEG resembling those seen in seizure patients. Yet the patient had no known seizures. A trial on an anticonvulsant produced a significant improvement, suggesting that the discharge has more handicapping effects than just seizures. This may be seen in temporal lobe seizure disorders, but it is not a frequent occurrence. When it does occur, the question arises whether the patient's discharges are really not producing any seizure symptoms or whether they are overlooked. The child may be hospitalized for a period of observation, but often a psychologist who is trained to watch the child and observe behaviors as well as test scores may pick up the elusive seizure symptoms that the medical staff and family have overlooked. She may be able to correlate the attack to a faltering, a pause, or a disturbance in the testing performance.

The length of a generalized seizure burst relates somewhat to symptoms. A generalized brain discharge lasting less than 3 seconds usually has minimum observable effect on the child's behavior problem. Discharges lasting from 3 to 5 seconds may be accompanied by a momentary pause in activities. A discharge lasting 5 to 7 seconds may present with a brief moment of confusion. A discharge of 10 or more seconds usually produces some type of recognizable seizure symptom. Spells lasting 30 seconds or more usually involve some type of obvious movement. Spells lasting 10 minutes or more, but not presenting as a clear-cut major motor convulsion, often are not seizures.

The epileptic child may have some problem in learning processing just before, during, and after a seizure. His thought processing may be slowed, distorted, or tenuous. The attack may wipe out immediate memories and dilute recent memories with old thoughts.

SPEECH PROBLEMS AND SEIZURES

Speech and language problems may be seen with obvious seizures or with patients with a left hemispheric disturbance, especially if it involves the left temporal lobe, with or without any psychomotor symptoms. The problem may be but another symptom of an underlying brain abnormality or it may be caused by subclinical seizure discharge.

Symptoms of an ongoing disturbance of speech and language, although varying from day to day, must be differentiated from the brief episodes of disturbed speech functions due to the actual seizure attack and from the aftereffects seen during the recovery period. In chronic speech and language problems there may be a deterioration in the clarity or the smooth flow of speech, in word selection, and in understanding or word order or word sounds when the patient tries to express his thoughts. The adult is more apt to talk excessively, to use trite or stereotyped phrases, or to repeat certain words, phrases, or sentences. The child may not show these symptoms. He does not confuse words of a similar nature as often as the adult does. His speech may be slow and stumbling, difficult to understand, or peppered with unexpected and sometimes peculiar word selections that are similar to, but not correct for, the idea. The child often shows more subtle signs of delayed or deviant development. He may not be able to speak or he may speak with a slow, labored, slurred, and often vague speech pattern, some of which is an attempt to compensate for his language difficulties. His speech may clear markedly for periods of time corresponding to the introduction of certain anticonvulsants or even a bout of illness. The opposite may also occur. Too often a physician tells the parents of a young child that he will probably grow out of his problem. This is not true. A child who has delayed speech or a deviation from normal significant enough to disturb the parents, frustrate the child, or be apparent to the physician should be referred for speech and language evaluation.

Speech and language problems may be due to an underlying brain lesion, such as a focal chronic virus infection, a tumor, or a vascular malformation. It may relate to an incompletely controlled seizure discharge or a drug reaction. Sometimes the seizures appear to be controlled but the speech problem persists. With an occasional patient, an increase or an alteration of the anticonvulsant within the normal therapeutic range may overcome the speech difficulties also. If the child has an active process of the brain, the speech may continue to deteriorate. However, if the seizures eventually improve or become controlled, the language function also may improve or recover. Usually there is a delay period. In an occasional patient the speech problem may develop prior to the seizure difficulties. A child with any type of speech problems may be at increased risk for problems in the processing of what he hears into what he says. This is a left hemispheric function. The child may also be a risk for having difficulties in reading by sounding out words. Early speech therapy may help overcome this future reading problem.

SPECIFIC LEARNING DISABILITIES

A specific learning disability is a block in learning in which one or more stages of the learning processes are significantly beneath the overall intellectual level, be it average, above average, or below average. This block is handicapping. It shows up as characteristic disorders in reading, writing, spelling, arithmetic, attention, coordination, listening, speech, remembering, understanding, or expression. Special terms, such as dyslexia (meaning abnormal reading), dysgraphia (abnormal writing), dyscalculia (abnormal math problem solving), or anarithmia (lack of arithmetic skills), are often used to describe learning disabilities seen in the classroom. However, these terms are not specific, since there are many types and patterns of dyslexia, dysgraphia, dyscalculia, etc. A dyslexic child may struggle to read. He may not be able to read up to his age or intellectual level. He may be able to read but he may not understand or recall what he reads. He may make peculiar or bizarre errors in his reading and often in his spelling. In general, epileptic children tend to be depressed in reading abilities, irrespective of their intellectual level. They may be below standard in other school skills also. In a rare patient, the act of reading itself may precipitate a seizure.

These reading, writing, spelling, and arithmetic problems, like other problems related to learning skills, are often due to a block in the processing of information in the mind. The type of block and the characteristic resultant errors in the school skills tend to relate to the location of the seizure focus in the brain.

There are a significant number of children in school who have such problems. This may be an inherited bad trait, passed on from parent to child, just as tone deafness often runs in families. It may be related to problems of birth, to chemical upsets in the body, to infections, to trauma, to tumors, or to seizures, as well as to the drugs used. A patient with focal seizures is especially prone to such difficulties. Even before the child's enrollment in school, the alert physician should be aware of what school skills should be monitored, especially when a seizure focus is identified.

Lateralization of Function

Each hemisphere has its own characteristic style of learning and consequent emotional reactions and behaviors. The left half of the brain, which is usually dominant, seems to process primarily speech and language, including understanding, remembering, and expression of words, phrases, and spoken ideas as well as writing. Other functions performed primarily by the left hemisphere include analysis, noting details, getting items in the correct order, judgments, noting time, and the process of calculation in math. Verbal skills include not only speech, but also memory, reasoning, verbal learning, and related verbalized emotions.

The right hemisphere seems most active in the processing of non-verbal, that is, non-language-dependent skills, including the recognition and remembering of geometric shapes, spatial arrangements and relationships, directions, right-left differentiation, and a sense of time. The right hemisphere helps people remember time and spatial patterns, such as melodies, faces, shapes, and forms.

Early Damage

If either hemisphere is damaged early in life, the other hemisphere may develop compensating functions, although they may not work as well as those of the originally intended brain half. For example, early damage to the left hemisphere may result in the development of most of the speech processes in the intact right hemisphere, but it will also result in lower intelligence. If the insult occurs in very early infancy, the onset and development of speech are often delayed. When it does appear, the speech may be disturbed in clarity, in smoothness, in quantity, in word selection, and in overall quality.

The patient who has early left hemisphere damage that involves hand usage may consequently develop as a left-handed person, since his left hand will work better than his right. A truly left-handed individual usually has a significant number of other family members who are left-handed, whereas the individual who has been forced to develop the use of his left side because of damage to the left hemisphere, and thus to the right body side, may not have a strong family history of left-handedness. The latter is an example of non-familial left-handedness, which is often accompanied by increased neurologic problems. Whenever the history reveals an individual to be left-handed, it should be determined whether there are other family members who are left-handed, i.e., whether there is familial left-handedness, or whether the individual, as the only left-hander, is more likely to be a non-familial left-handed individual.

Focal Seizures — Specific Learning Disabilities

The side of the seizure and the location of the discharge may relate to specific types of learning risks, which in turn may result in emotional and behavioral problems.

Frontal Lobe Seizure Foci People with frontal lobe abnormalities may also have difficulties with independent work efforts, especially those tasks that depend on developing one answer as a base to the next step. This is especially true if the right frontal lobe is significantly disturbed. A left frontal lobe involvement is more apt to disturb the smooth flow of spontaneous speech. The frontal lobes are not common sites for seizure foci as compared to the frequent temporal lobe foci, with the exception of the motor strip.

Left Temporal Lobe Foci Temporal lobe seizures differ in the types of associated learning disturbances, depending on whether the overall problem is a left or a right temporal lobe syndrome. Left temporal lobe seizures appear to be more common and often of earlier onset than right temporal lobe seizures. Language and verbal skills as well as related reasoning and verbal learning processes are affected. The person is apt to have problems recognizing and remembering what he hears. He may have problems with rote memory, in remembering words and names, math tables, rhymes, prayers, addresses, or phone numbers. Sometimes he recalls a similar but incorrect word, and this confusion will show up in his understanding, his speech, or his written efforts.

The child with a left temporal lobe disturbance may have problems both in reading and later in spelling. Phonetic approaches, such as blending sounds together into words, may be difficult for him. He has problems sounding out words. He may confuse similar sounds or words. Sometimes he gets the sounds or the letters in the wrong order. These problems carry over to his speech and spelling as well as to his reading. He cannot rely on basic spelling rules to help him since he may also have problems remembering them.

Left hemispheric seizure patients, and especially left temporal lobe patients, seem to be especially prone to reading problems. Intelligence testing comparisons of verbal and performance skills may not indicate what the problem is. Boys seem to be more at risk than girls. Unlike phenobarbital, when Mysoline, Zarontin, or Dilantin is used as the only controlling anticonvulsant, it seems to increase the risk for learning problems.

Math problems usually are apparent by the time the child reaches the third grade, if not earlier. The child may confuse or not recognize what operations the signs tell him to do, such as addition, subtraction, multiplication, or division. He may subtract larger numbers from smaller numbers. He may carry over the last number of the problem as the answer (this mistake is a form of perseveration). He may write numbers literally. For example, when told to write 164, he may write 100, 60, and 4, and often places the comma place markings incorrectly in 4-digit or higher numbers.

Right Temporal Lobe Foci If the seizure problem involves the right temporal lobe or adjacent brain areas, the child may have problems recognizing what he sees or non-language patterns that he hears. He may have problems remembering and recognizing shapes, patterns, and forms. Such problems are often referred to as visuospatial difficulties, visual/motor problems, or perceptual (motor) problems. The child tends to have problems recognizing familiar words when he sees them. He may even have problems recognizing letters and numbers. In reading or writing he may reverse, invert, or twist the letters around in his mind. In spelling, he may add letters, omit them, or sometimes double or even triple up a letter. Sometimes he fuses two letters together and sometimes he devises new letters. His writing tends to be very sloppy, with blotches and extra markings. His letters may vary in size, shape, form, and tilt; often he writes or prints with erratic spacing and little attention to the paper lines. Similarly, in math he may miss significant details, such as the operation signs. Sometimes he confuses the math columns and adds, subtracts, or multiplies from one column to the next. He may have problems with borrowing or carrying.

Such perceptual problems often result in clumsiness and a poor sense of left-right, directions, and time, as well as problems in table manners (spilling), sports (clumsy), housekeeping (overlooks obvious items), and in learning to sight read music. He may have problems recognizing social cues on other people's faces, resulting in disturbed social relationships. In reacting to his difficulties he may become quite rigid and adherent to set schedules, going to pieces when the unexpected happens. In left and right temporal lobe seizure patients there appear to be fewer risks for a gross visuospatial problem than there are for auditory processing deficits, as are seen with left temporal lobe seizures of early onset. However, subtle disturbances may still exist. Visual perception problems are the most common type of learning disability identified by present means.

Bilateral Temporal Lobe Foci If the onset of seizures occurs before the child is five years of age and appears in both temporal lobes, the child is at a greater risk for a combination of both auditory-to-vocal and visual-to-motor processing deficits, resulting in a lowered intelligence. He may also have difficulties with memory. Often inattentiveness and distractability, on-and-off learning, and incomplete work efforts are noted.

If surgery is performed for seizures and both inner surfaces of the temporal lobe (which contain an important structure, the hippocampus) are removed, the patient suffers a severe memory problem. He may not be able to remember what he has just seen or heard or what he was just doing if his attention is interrupted. However, his intelligence and his speech may remain intact, since he can rely on previously stored knowledge. Bilateral destruction of this important area may occur in the infant due to a lack of oxygen, low blood sugar levels, brain swelling, or poor blood flow to the brain. This damage not only causes seizures but also may produce marked disturbances in memory. The child may not be able to remember something long enough to learn it. Since he has no past memories to rely on, he may seem to be severely retarded. The optimal teaching method for such a child is to approach him as if he had a severe memory and distractability problem, i.e., a type of learning disability.

Early Signs

These learning problem risks may show up as poor sucking and feeding in the neonate, as crawling and coordination problems in the infant, or as speech problems in the toddler. The preschool child may be slow to learn his numbers, his letters, nursery rhymes, names, or addresses. He might not like to color, to cut, or to read. He may be slowed and confused at tying, buttoning, or dressing. He may be delayed in telling time.

In the first grade the child is most apt to have reading problems. Because of his frustrations he may be mistakenly branded as hyperkinetic. By third grade, spelling and math problems may become major difficulties. If he is not given appropriate help, by the second decade of life he may become so frustrated that he begins to act out his frustrations. He may give up and do nothing, attempt to run away or to avoid efforts, become angry and aggressive, become anxious and develop physical complaints, or become discouraged even to the point of attempting suicide. Delinquency is not an uncommon consequence of untreated learning disabilities.

Diagnosis

A patient with a focal seizure disorder, especially if it appears before six years of age and most especially if there is a known or suspected etiology, is at risk for a learning disability. The types of drugs used, the degree of seizure control, and the previous help and handling also affect this. Realizing these significant risks, the physician should be on guard and looking for early signs of problems so that he can refer the patient for adequate identification and remediation early, before the complicating emotional reactions to frustration emerge.

DEPRESSED AND DETERIORATING INTELLIGENCE

Seizures themselves do not lead to a decrease in intelligence unless they are frequent, prolonged, or severe. Learning problems and seizures may be symptoms of underlying brain disturbances. Epileptic patients who do not have known brain damage tend to fall into the normal range of intelligence. However, they do tend to cluster toward the lower range of normal. There also appears to be greater frequency of more subtle learning problems. This may be more common to the lower socioeconomic level, perhaps due to the lack of stimulating activities.

A lower intelligence does not prevent the child from having a specific learning disability. Such a child may be more at a risk for having an imbalanced learning process, especially if the depressed intelligence is due to some brain insult. Often the distribution of the insult to the brain is uneven. Consequently the effects on learning and the resultant learning processes would also seem likely to be equally uneven. Some causes of retardation may be no more than a severe learning disability in the early stages of learning. This may be accentuated by the consequent development of frustration and giving up. Severely distorted learning processing of all channels, but especially of the handling of speech, with confusing, labored, disorganized processes, may even be a major factor in autism, which has a common finding of a severe impairment of language development, intelligence, and both social and behavioral interactions. In some individuals the autistic symptoms and the left temporal lobe seizure consequence may be somewhat similar. Sometimes treating various types of retardation and autism as if they were severe learning processing problems can result in striking improvement. As autism and seizures have a more than expected overlay in the frequency of presentation in the young child, there may be a relationship. In general, lowered intelligence and psychiatric problems are common associates in both the normal and the epileptic population. Some factors associated with the retardation include frequent seizures, missed or unrecognized convulsive attacks, and early onset of seizures. Patients with neonatal seizures, infantile myoclonic spasms, atypical absence attacks (especially with a slow spike/wave EEG pattern), and temporal lobe seizures (especially left) appear to be at increased risk for relative mental retardation.

Causes of Depressed or Deteriorating Intelligence

Intelligence problems may relate to the underlying brain problem that also causes the seizure. They may also relate to the age of onset, frequent recurrence, prolonged attacks, or the drugs used. Other problems, such as specific learning difficulties, frustration and discouragement, or behavior disturbances may inhibit the development of learning. The attitudes and management of the patient at home and at school are important factors influencing the development of normal or abnormal learning.

Intellectual Failing

In a significant number of seizure patients there is a falling off of intelligence, emotions, or behavior. This may be due to the effects of repeated seizures, to chronic drug usage or an abnormal drug reaction, or to the underlying brain problem. Drugs, especially Dilantin and Mysoline, may be associated with such a deterioration of function. Changing from a "problem" drug to another, less bothersome one, such as phenobarbital, frequently, but not always, may overcome this, if the problem is caught early enough. This is why the patient's function, as well as his seizure control status and his medication tolerance, must be monitored closely and frequently.

Some patients with repeated seizures may begin to deteriorate. Animal studies have shown that, when seizures are created in the temporal lobes, after 25 or 30 seizures the nerve cells in the temporal lobes begin to die off on their own. In humans operated on for temporal lobe seizures, examination of the brain tissue has shown nerve cells in different stages of cell death. This finding suggests a need for an intensive effort to control all seizures.

Children with known brain lesions, with early onset of seizures, and with generalized motor or temporal lobe seizures seem to be at risk for intellectual deterioration. However, in light of the numerous potential causes, careful observation and detection of early signs of deterioration may allow the physician to intervene and possibly prevent permanent damage.

PLACEMENT

Most children can and should be placed in an appropriate learning situation, not a home-based teaching program. A few patients may be so severely handicapped that they require institutional care. These are usually children that show no potential for communicating by any means in order to learn or are so severely handicapped that they require special helps not available in the community but available in a progressive institution. No patient with any potential should be denied an opportunity to an education just because he has seizures. He needs to go to school. Epileptic children need the opportunity to develop social skills as well as to learn. This is why a classroom placement is most important. Nearly 1 of every 4 epileptic children may require specialized educational services, be it special education for the retarded, the learning disabled, the emotionally disturbed, the gifted, the crippled, or individuals with some other handicap. Appropriate placement may be limited by the lack of a reasonable seizure control, which aggravates already present problems with school attitudes. Yet an alert and interested teacher often is the best monitor of the child's function, provided she has the support of and open communication with the physician.

Right to an Education

If a child is not achieving up to expectation, the school should try to discover why. This should lead to various tests of intellectual and academic function. When such tests do not indicate the reason, the school authorities may tend to blame the problem on behavior. Misbehavior in class is most often a symptom of frustration, not the cause of learning problems.

Parents have various rights regarding their child's education. Parents have the right to receive written notice of any efforts to alter a child's school program or any refusal to make a needed change. Parents have the right to give or withhold permission for the child to be tested, evaluated by specialists, or placed in a specific program. Parents have the right to see and examine all school records that relate to the identification of any problems, the evaluation and testing, and the placement of the child. If a parent feels the records are inaccurate or misleading, that parent may request that they be removed from the child's files. Once records have been removed from the files, they may not be used in planning for the child's placement. The parent has the right to request an impartial hearing to protest any decision regarding identifying problems, evaluating needs, or placement of the child. If the first protest is not successful, an appeal can be made to the state Department of Education or even to courts if necessary.

If the child seems to have special needs, the parent should notify the school about the handicap. Usually the superintendent or director of specialized educational services should be contacted. The school is obligated to identify and serve all children with handicaps. If a child is found to be eligible for specialized educational services, a meeting that includes the parents must be held within 30 days to prepare an individualized educational program. This applies not just to younger children but also to adolescents. Many states provide by law for special programs beginning at age 3.

Parents should attempt to work with the teacher, the principal, the specialist, and the superintendent whenever possible. Parents should be allies and advocates rather than adversaries of the professionals whenever possible.

Parents can request an evaluation or a re-evaluation whenever they are dissatisfied with their child's placement, especially if the placement is based on incomplete, old, or inaccurate information or the program does not seem satisfactory. All requests should be put in writing. If a vital discussion occurs on the phone, a letter should be written to confirm the finding. Copies of all letters and requests should be kept on file by the parents to document what has been done. The file should contain test results, professional reports, the parents' notations, reports and memos from school, letters and responses from school officials, and, whenever possible, copies of pertinent state and federal laws.

Parents should be sure that the testing evaluation was complete and was performed by a team of specialists who covered all pertinent aspects of the child's needs. Evaluation should include a complete physical examination, as well as testing, in order to make sure that any contributing physical defect has been noted. Often the labels used to identify a child tend to indicate his handicaps, i.e., what he cannot do, they do not indicate his potential and strengths. However, strengths *should* be included in the evaluation. Parents also should discuss their observations of the child's weaknesses, strengths, behaviors, and needs with the team. Parents should be a vital component of the team.

Parents should ask what test or tests are to be given, what the tests will tell, and why they are given, before they permit testing to begin. Be sure that the testing does not discriminate in any way, be it in language or style (such as visual tests for the visually handicapped, or tests dependent on hearing for the deaf, or language-dependent tests for learning disabled children). The family has the right to expect that the testing, the reason for testing, the results and their meanings be explained in simple, clear terms, not in technical terms. The family should obtain a copy of the testing for their own files.

The goal of identification and evaluation is to place the child in the best type of educational setting. Placement is based on the development of an individualized education program (IEP). Legally, the parent must be a part of the planning team that develops the IEP. The planning team also includes the child's teacher and a representative of the school system as well as various specialists. The school is responsible for contacting the parents to arrange for the IEP developmental meetings to be held at a time convenient for the parents. An IEP must be developed for every child who is eligible for a special education placement. The parents should be prepared for the meeting. An up-to-date file that includes the school records, including results of the most recent evaluations, is a great help. The parents may wish to bring a helper to serve as an advocate. Some members of pertinent advocacy and parent groups are willing to do this. The parents should have a clear idea of what is needed for the child. This idea should be backed up by substantiating professional opinions. The parents have the right to ask the professional to accompany them to the meeting. Parents must realize that a diagnostic report, although it is a great help, may not be completely correct. If there are any questionable areas, they should be discussed.

The parent should consider what placement may be best for the child. Classes chosen by labels (such as blind, retarded, physically handicapped) tend to be stigmatizing but may offer the concentrated services needed by a severely handicapped child. Mainstreaming a child into a regular classroom with individualized special helps given to his needs may be less stigmatizing and more normalizing, and therefore more desirable, unless it means he won't get the intensive help needed. The parents should be aggressive yet agreeable, assertive yet not antagonistic as the IEP is developed. An open-minded approach, using persuasion and persistent questioning, is more apt to lead to a mutual understanding than an angry, demanding confrontation.

The parents also should inspect the classroom and its environment. The teacher is the most important component. A good teacher is more important than the type of class or the place of the class. The school cannot exclude children with physical handicaps because of an architectural barrier, such as stairs, since the law requires that school facilities be made accessible and safe. Special adaptations may need to be made so that services are available to all students that need them.

When an IEP is finally developed, the parents should receive a copy in writing. They should review the IEP carefully, to be sure that it contains clear prescriptions both for the handling of immediate problems as well as for long-term objectives. It should spell out the length of time to be spent at each stage and what services are needed and must be provided for achievement of the child's goals. It should be clearly written so that the family can understand it. If there are any doubts, the family should take the IEP to consultants to help determine if it is good or if it contains areas of concern yet to be clarified or developed. The parents should be persistent in seeking appropriate vocational education in their child's IEP if this is indicated. They should be firm about important concerns, but they should still be ready to compromise.

If the parents are dissatisfied with the decisions of the school, they may seek additional testing or consultation. The school may agree to this and bear the expense; if it does not, then the parents can request a hearing, presided over by an official who is impartial, i.e., not employed by the school district or involved in the education of the child. The parents may also obtain testing at their own expense if the school refuses to do the testing. If the hearing decides such testing is indicated, the school must then pay for the testing; however, if the hearing feels that the school was correct in its assumption that testing was not needed, the parents must pay for the tests. The parents can and often should be accompanied by a representative of the advocacy group (see Chapter 14) and, if it is felt necessary, by a legal counsel, such as an advocate or lawyer familiar with the educational law. If the hearing at the local level does not support the parents' claims, they may go on to hearings at the state level or even appeal in court. A hearing in the district must be held within 45 days of the request; a hearing at the state Department of Education level must be reviewed within 30 days. The state advocacy program may be a valuable asset (see Chapter 14).

Once the child is placed in a satisfactory program, the parents are not finished with their efforts. They should become involved with the teacher, working closely with her in order to share concerns, needs, and approaches, and to learn how efforts might be improved at home to help the school. Sometimes the teacher may need and desire more understanding about the handicap. She may be uneasy because she is caught between parental pressure and administrative admonitions without any training to understand or to cope with what she is mandated to do. The parents should be sure that a formal evaluation of the child's progress occurs annually and that this is satisfactory and up to the mutually agreed upon expectations outlined in the IEP. If an annual evaluation is not being done, the school should determine why.

Parents all too often leave planning for their epileptic child up to others: they tend to give up, to accept inferior programs, or to allow their feelings to be overlooked. This places a smaller load on the school, but the child suffers. The parents should feel involved; they should not be awed by the professionals. In turn, the professionals should encourage parental involvement, since everyone should be attending the planning meeting for the mutual purpose of aiding the child. The plans should cover not just education, but also social interactions, vocational preparation, and recreation. Often the parents feel powerless and alone when faced with the bureaucracy of the school system. Banding together in organizations of parents and families of handicapped individuals helps to support the parents in their pursuit of needed services for their children. Parents' organizations can also help make the school system aware of the needs of the handicapped.

CONCLUSION

When a diagnosis of a seizure disorder is made, the physician must consider how the attacks may affect the child's learning and behavioral development as well as their impact on the family's relationships and attitudes. Merely attaching labels and prescribing pills is insufficient. Frequent follow-up monitoring may catch early adverse changes or emerging problems before they become significant or severe. The physician needs to ask about school or work performance, behavioral problems, and emotional difficulties, just as he asks about the seizure controls, drug reactions, and any illnesses. He must treat the whole patient, not just the seizures. A whole-person management approach often not only helps to lessen the major problems of learning and emotional difficulties, but also improves anticonvulsant compliance, resulting in improved seizure control.

REFERENCES AND SUGGESTED READING

(The) Commission for the Control of Epilepsy and Its Consequences. 1977-78. Plan for Nationwide Action on Epilepsy. U.S. Dept. of Health, Education and Welfare, National Institutes of Health, DHEW Publication No. (NIH) 78-279, Office of Scientific and Health Reports, NINCDS-NIH, Bethesda, Md. 4 Volumes; especially helpful is H. R. Myklebust, Educational Problems of the Child with Epilepsy, Vol. II, pp. 474-490.

Dikmen, S., and C. G. Matthews. 1977. Effect of major motor seizure frequency upon cognitive-intellectual functions in adults. Epilepsia 18:21-29.

Dikmen, S., C. G. Matthews, and J. P. Harley. 1975. The effect of early versus late onset of major motor epilepsy upon cognitive-intellectual performance: Epilepsia 16:73-81.

Dikmen, S., C. G. Matthews, and J. P. Harley. 1977. Effect of early versus late onset of major motor epilepsy on cognitive-intellectual performance: Further considerations. Epilepsia 18:31-36.

Epilepsy Foundation of America. 1975. Basic Statistics on the Epilepsies. F. A. Davis Co., Philadelphia. 155 pp.

Forster, C. 1977. Aphasia and seizure disorders in childhood. In: J. K. Penry (ed.), Epilepsy, The Eighth International Symposium, pp. 305-366. Raven Press, New York.

Lou, H. C., S. Brandt, and P. Brandt. 1977. Progressive aphasia and epilepsy with a self-limited course. In: J. K. Penry (ed.), Epilepsy, The Eighth International Symposium, pp. 295-304. Raven Press, New York.

McIntyre, M., P. B. Pritchard III, and C. T. Lombroso. 1976. Left and right temporal lobe epileptics: A controlled investigation of some psychological differences. Epilepsia 17:377-386.

Mellor, D. H., and I. Lowit. 1977. A study of intellectual function in children with epilepsy attending ordinary schools. In: J. K. Penry (ed.), Epilepsy, The Eighth International Symposium, pp. 291-294. Raven Press, New York.

Ounsted, C., J. Lindsay, and R. Norman. 1966. Biologic Factors in Temporal Lobe Epilepsy. Clinics of Developmental Medicine No. 22. Wm. Heinemann Medical Books Ltd., London, 135 pp.

Reitan, R. M. 1947. Psychological testing of epileptic patients. In: O. Magnus and A. M. Lorentz de Haas (eds.), The Epilepsies, Vol. 15, Chapter 9, pp. 189-218. P. J. Vincken and G. W. Bruyn (eds.), Handbook of Clinical Neurology. Elsevier-North Holland Publishing Company, New York.

Rodin, E. A., M. Katz, and K. Lennox. 1976. Differences between patients with temporal lobe seizures and those with other forms of seizure attacks. Epilepsia 17:313-320.

Rodin, E., P. Rennick, R. Dennerll, and Y. Lin. 1972. Vocational and educational problems of epileptic patients. Epilepsia 13:149-160.

Scheiber, B. (ed.) 1976. You have rights — Use them! In: Closer Look, Special issue of Fall, 1977. National Information Center for the Handicapped, Box 1492, Washington, D.C.

14
RESTRICTIONS AND RESOURCES

The epileptic patient is continually haunted by his capricious convulsive disorder, which, without any real warning, can cruelly interrupt his activities. During an attack, the patient is helpless, non-functioning, and totally dependent upon others. Between attacks he can function normally, but society tends to limit his functioning.

SPORTS ACTIVITIES

Exercise is good for all people, including epileptics. It may even reduce seizure frequency. Competitive or individual sports may allow the frustrated individual to release some of his pent-up anger resulting from his seizure problem. Very often the individual is over-restricted. The parents fear that the child might hurt himself or even be killed by a seizure during athletic competition. They fear that the excitement or bodily trauma may bring on an attack. The school fears that the epileptic athlete may be injured during an attack and they might be held liable. The coach, the teammates, and even the patient himself may fear that the game may be lost because of an attack. The patient also fears the embarrassment of a seizure in public.

The excitement of the event and the stresses of the sport may trigger a seizure, but restricting the patient from such activities may lead only to denial and rebellion. The patient's disappointment may be expressed by erratic intake of his medicine, which consequently may cause his seizures to become more frequent, and his behavior to deteriorate. However, if he is allowed to participate appropriately in sports, the patient may become careful in his care and medicine intake in order to safeguard his continued participation.

Usually little restriction, if any, is needed in sports. With some uncontrolled seizure disorders, the choice may be between a contact and a noncontact sport, between a competitive and a non-competitive effort, or between individual and team sports activities. Tying together sports participation, good seizure care, and satisfactory school performance as a related responsibility of the patient may achieve maximum benefits in all areas.

OTHER ACTIVITIES

The question of the amount of restriction that should be placed on the patient in other activities arises. These activities include riding bicycles, horses, or motorcycles, climbing trees or to heights, using power tools (such as drills, lawnmowers, power saws, etc.), or going on outings. The degree of restraint, if any, and the number of precautions relate to the state of control over the seizures. If the seizures are completely uncontrolled, the patient should avoid activities that represent a realistic danger should a seizure occur during the activity. The patient should be allowed to participate in other activities only with certain common-sense precautions. If the seizures are in the process of being controlled with active changing of medicines, it is probably wise to impose some temporary restrictions and precautions, but the patient should realize that restrictions are only *temporary* and that they will be reduced or stopped when control is reached. With controlled seizures, minimum if any restrictions need be imposed, depending on the length of the seizure control state.

The major consideration in deciding what is a reasonable and proper restraint is to what degree risks exist for potential injury should a seizure occur during the activity. This means how high off the ground, how fast moving, or how much alone the patient may be during the activity that might be interrupted by a seizure. Generally, heights and fast speeds should be avoided, especially if the seizures are not controlled. If the seizure patient is with someone else who could help if an attack occurred, many activities (for example, swimming) can be allowed that otherwise would not be advisable if the patient is alone. Often such activities should not be undertaken by one person alone anyway. The choice of safe areas for riding rather than busy roadways or the selection of power machinery with automatic safety shut-off switches may allow a greater degree of normal activities.

The tendency is toward an unreasonable amount of restriction and precautions. An epileptic patient, realizing how hesitantly permission is given and how quickly it is withdrawn, is more apt to avoid any careless accidents than the average person. Thus his risks may be less, not greater, than others'. A responsible patient may be allowed more privileges. This strengthens the patient's cooperation in management of his seizures and his life, leading to improved seizure control and fewer emotional problems. Slight risks in certain situations may be worth the overall benefits.

DRIVING RESTRICTIONS

The restrictions against driving placed on the epileptic adolescent affect prestige, dating, transportation, and employment. The teenager dreams of his first car and often is crushed by being forbidden to drive. Yet he must be truthful in his driver's license application. He has two hurdles to face: getting the license and obtaining auto collision insurance. If he hides his seizures and subsequently is involved in an accident, he is apt to find himself both uninsured and judged liable for the accident no matter who was at fault.

States vary in the restrictions they place on an epileptic's driving. The ideal rule might be that the seizures be controlled for a minimum of 3 to 6 months before the patient can be issued a restricted license with periodic review. If the seizures occur infrequently and only at night in sleep, the license may only restrict the patient from driving at night. Once two years of total control have been reached, the patient may be issued a permanent license, although periodic medical re-examinations may still be desirable. When the patient has been off anticonvulsant therapy for three years without any recurrence of the attacks, there should be no further restrictions.

The laws on driving vary from state to state. These can be obtained from the State Department of Motor Vehicles or some similar state agency. In some states, the application must be accompanied by a physician's statement certifying the duration of the medical care, the length of time of the seizure control, the medications used, and the physician's opinions regarding the risks of a seizure breakthrough.

It is sad but true that for some patients driving must be considered a luxury, not a right. Any patient depending on medication for seizure control should consider what would happen if a seizure occurs. He should plan his lifestyle accordingly. It is probably advisable for him to live near a means of public transportation, within reasonable walking distance of his job and any shopping centers. Thus if he should have recurring seizures and lose his licence, he will not be as handicapped as the individual who finds himself trapped away from any means of getting to work, to school, or to other facilities. He may become unemployed and dependent on others for essentials. The patient who has not planned ahead must search for an alternate means of transportation, such as a car pool, if he is to be able to get around.

In modern society, the driver's license has become a vital means of identification. The seizure patient may not qualify for this needed identification under normal circumstances. However, in many states the Department of Motor Vehicles or of Highways or Transportation will issue a special license that will serve to identify the patient although it still restricts him from driving.

INSURANCE

It may be very difficult, very expensive, and often seem impossible for the epileptic person to obtain any type of insurance. Special problems exist with life, health, and car insurance. He may have to pay much higher premiums yet still find major restrictions within his policy.

Sometimes a child can be maintained on his family's insurance policy on into adulthood. A family is wise to obtain as much insurance on the child as possible as part of a family group plan, so that the child can carry this over to adulthood. Sometimes the epileptic employee can obtain insurance through his company's group policies. He should get all the coverage he can and maintain it even if he changes jobs. The Epilepsy Foundation of America offers a national insurance program as an alternative or supplement.

DATING, MARRIAGE, AND FAMILY

If a date is based on simple friendship, it is a matter of choice whether the epileptic tells his date of his problem. However, if the relationship begins to become serious, the partner should be told. A strong relationship is based on trust and openness. Withholding facts only leads to mistrust, resentment, and possible grounds for future break-up of the marriage. The epileptic individual lives in fear that his secret will be discovered. In a successful marriage, the spouses must be completely open and accepting of each other without reservation. The couple should seriously discuss the anticipated frustrations, social restrictions, employment difficulties, their feelings, the management of the seizures, the effects of seizures on the relationship, and the risk of seizures in the offspring. All too often there is the tendency to continue to hide these concerns rather than to face them, even after marriage. A serious date or a spouse may appear most understanding and accepting but still be struggling with acceptance.

The concern regarding future offspring often is a major question. Although the risks are low, the chances of having a child with seizures may be greater if the seizures are of no known cause or appear in other family members, and especially if the history of seizures is strong on both sides of the family or in both spouses themselves. If only one of the partners has a seizure problem or a positive family history of seizures, he may feel guilty and responsible if his child develops seizures. This is especially true if the probabilities have not been discussed. Even if neither parent has a history of epilepsy, the development of a seizure problem in the child may cause parents to reconsider whether they should have any further children.

PROBLEMS OF EMPLOYMENT

A significant number of capable seizure patients are underemployed or frankly unemployed. This is more due to the attitudes of society than to the disability of the patient. Even a significantly handicapped epileptic patient can become a productive wage-earner if adequate provisions are developed.

Regular Employment

Many firms refuse to hire a known epileptic patient. The applicant may find that he must state on the application forms that he has epilepsy. He is faced with the choice of whether to hide this and face future firing, or to be honest and consequently not hired. Sometimes this information may be given in confidence rather than on the form. A majority of employers state that they are willing to consider an epileptic candidate for a position but in practice only a minority of employers will actually hire such an applicant.

Attitude The firm's supervisors and other employees fear working with an epileptic individual because they fear the stigma of epilepsy. They are concerned that he will not carry his share of the job load. They do not know what to do if they are faced with a seizure on the job; consequently they prefer not to be subjected to the problem.

The potential employer fears that his insurance rates will go up because of the individual's seizures leading to an increased accident rate. He fears that the epileptic employee will be excessively absent due to his seizures. He does not want to have to deal with the reactions of his other employees.

The epileptic applicant does not improve his chances if he seeks a job with a chip on his shoulder. Attitudes such as "The world owes me a job because I am epileptic," "You must hire me because I am a handicapped person," or "If you don't hire me, you are discriminating against handicapped individuals and especially against epileptic citizens," or the crusader who considers himself hired only to spend his time educating others about epilepsy rather than working, often result in the individual not being hired or being fired at the first opportunity. Such attitudes do more to discourage than to encourage an employer to hire any epileptic candidates.

Employers tend to reject the applicant because he is felt to be different, dangerous to himself and to others, unable to produce consistently, disturbing to employee morale, or possessing an undesirable attitude, the latter being the only valid reason. The reasons given for not hiring are that the job opening has been filled or the applicant does not meet the requirements of the position. The employer to be commended is the one that makes an effort to adapt a position or creates a new position for a trial period for a reasonable applicant even if he has reservations, providing he has the need for such an employee.

Schools are hesitant to hire epileptic staff people because they fear that a seizure in the classroom may disturb the children and cause consequent complaints from parents.

Myths and Truths The major problem is to convince the employer and his employees that an epileptic applicant can be reliable, efficient, productive, and safe as an employee. An additional problem may be to convince the applicant to become a desirable employee and not to be an irritating epileptic crusader.

Most of the employer's fears prove unfounded. The absentee record of an epileptic employee due to health and seizure problems may be only slightly higher than that of the average employee. A day or so of lost time because of epilepsy is insignificant compared to the seven to ten days lost due to other illnesses by the average employee.

The safety record of a properly placed epileptic employee is usually better than the average employee's record. In those industries willing to hire epileptics, insurance rates and compensation costs have been reduced because of a good safety record. The job performance tends to be satisfactory, if not above average. The epileptic patient is in a critical spotlight and he knows it. He cannot afford any further problems. Consequently he may try harder to be extra-productive, fully efficient, present, and performing with extreme care to avoid any accidents, absences, or incompleteness.

Proper Job Selection If the patient's seizures would at best be only partially controlled, certain job situations probably would best be avoided. Jobs that create an excess of tension and emotional stress, those with irregular hours, those with environmental stimuli known to aggravate the patient's seizures, and those that might be excessively risky should a seizure occur should be avoided. Risky jobs include driving, working in high places, working near large or deep bodies of water, and working around heavy machinery, electrical circuits, flames, heat, or corrosive materials. A patient may be restricted from obtaining jobs to which he must drive unless he can find an alternative means of transportation. Solitary jobs, such as guard duty, may not be desirable if the seizures are not controlled.

Sometimes a modification in the job or making allowance for certain restrictions, made on an individual basis, may enable the patient to accept a job. The modification needed depends on the seizure pattern, the degree of control, the demands of the job, and the cooperation of the employer. A patient who has seizures only at night or associated with sleep is at minimum risk for a daytime job; he should avoid jobs that are irregular in hours or that interfere with a regular sleep routine. A patient who routinely experiences a significant warning-aura may be able to seek out safety before the main attack occurs; he may be able to handle some jobs ordinarily not advisable for the usual epileptic individual. The employment situation may be altered to make some jobs more available. Pairing employees in a "buddy" system or altering the machinery, such as the incorporation of an automatic shut-off switch that deactivates the machine if hand-pressure is released, may open up further job possibilities.

Preparing the Patient

There are many job opportunities for a majority of epileptic individuals if they are ready for them. The patient needs to be guided toward these jobs, depending on his interests, skills, and abilities. Such preparation should not be put off until the individual is at least 16 years old and eligible for a vocational preparatory program. It should be begun by at least the beginning of the second decade of life. Part of this preparation involves the school and part involves actively working with the parents and the patient.

Academic Preparation The school needs to prepare the patient in three ways. He will need the basic educational skills to subsist in daily life situations, such as shopping, measuring (as in cooking and carpentry), handling of money, and other basics. He also needs the basic academic skills required in his anticipated vocation, especially if he has a learning handicap, as frequently occurs with seizures. This includes developing basic reading skills and a vocationally related sight vocabulary as well as the practical math skills he will need. Finally, the school should supply an accepting, open environment in which the child can develop his social skills.

Medical Preparation Some patients may have the potential for an acceptable job placement if the seizure control can be improved and if any unwanted side effects of the drug can be overcome. A job placement may need to be postponed temporarily while this is accomplished. Ideally, vocational preparation and medical care can be combined so that there will be no need for any last-minute delays.

Vocational Preparation Some patients may be medically ready but not vocationally prepared for employment. The individual does not know what he can do, how to prepare himself to work, or how to look for a job. Such preparation should be a vital component of a good management program.

If social and emotional problems emerge as a block to employment, the patient needs counseling in order to understand himself and how his attitudes and actions affect others. He must accept the attitudes of others rather than continuing to confront, resist, and antagonize them. He must build up his own self-concept and confidence yet he still must realistically accept his restrictions and limitations. He must expect acceptance on the basis of what he is, not on the basis of his handicap. If the individual cannot accept his own epilepsy, he should not expect others to.

Emphasis must be placed on good medical management of the seizure problem. This is the patient's responsibility, not anyone else's. Good management includes regular medicine intake, regular medical check-ups, and close cooperation with his physician. He must realize that the medicine is not a cure, it only suppresses the seizure tendency if he takes it regularly. It cannot be over-emphasized that erratic intake leads to poor seizure control, which may interfere with efforts to find and keep employment. A patient who achieves the independence of employment may also begin to feel independent of any doctor telling him what he should or should not do, and he may begin neglecting medical check-ups and feeling autonomous about his drug regimen. He may return only when necessary to obtain a prescription renewal. He may begin to experiment with his medicines himself rather than following the prescribed instructions. Although the patient needs to have his independence encouraged and his sense of responsibility for his own seizure management established, he still also needs to maintain good medical care and support.

Former employment records and job interview experiences, both successful and unsuccessful, should be reviewed. With the patient's permission, former employers and potential employers should be contacted. Strengths and weaknesses should be identified. The patient may desperately need training in how to interview for a job.

Vocational counselors also may obtain specific tests as well as conduct interviews with the patient in order to determine specific interests and potential skills. Based on this information, the counselor can help develop the client's potential, can identify job possibilities, and can steer the client toward an appropriate application. It remains the duty of the client to make the actual application.

Employer Preparation The counselor must also work closely with a potential employer and, if allowed, his employees, educating them about what epilepsy is and what it isn't. This includes basic management methods in handling an actual attack. Some corporations require basic first-aid training of their employees. This is to be encouraged. However, the first aid for epilepsy may be superficial and the methods used may be outdated. Offering good modern training assistance may benefit both the industry and its potential employees. The counselor needs to impress the employer with the potential capabilities of the epileptic individual. He may even welcome ideas for improving programs, especially if these are at a low cost or no cost.

The National Association of Epilepsy Executives is a growing group of employers engaged in developing awareness of the needs as well as the employability of epileptic individuals by businesses. Employment service information and wage data are also being accumulated.

As in many other businesses, civil service jobs may require that the patient state that he has epilepsy. This information can be given in confidence. The question on the application regarding epilepsy need not be answered, although the blank almost answers itself. If a job application is accompanied by a physician's statement that the seizures are under reliable control, the employer may be more willing to consider the application for employment. Some government agencies have a special handicapped program in which the severely disabled applicant is given a three- or four-month trial period on the job, to prove his abilities and simultaneously to gain job experience. The final decision is then made regarding permanent employment. Sometimes the employing agency is impressed with the record but dubious about certain aspects of the performance. The employing agency may be able to adapt the job so as to conform to the skills of the applicant. Many of the government agencies have removed epilepsy from the group of severe disabilities. Consequently it is left up to the epileptic individual to prove that his epilepsy is or is not a severe disability, if he is to be allowed the trial.

This is an example of the term "epilepsy" serving as a benefit rather than a stigma. Too much effort has been made to hide the term under other alternate terms, avoiding the word so vehemently that the use becomes more handicapping than the meaning. It is probably best to bring epilepsy out into the open, working to change public attitudes rather than to alter the word.

Federal and State Programs

Under the Vocational Rehabilitation Act of 1973 and the Amendment of 1974, there are specific sections forbidding the discrimination against handicaps in hiring and requiring the development of affirmative action plans toward the hiring of disabled individuals. This law applies to any state, public, or private firm that receives federal monies. The basic statute states that no individual who is otherwise qualified can, solely because of his handicap, be excluded from participating in or receiving the benefits of, or be discriminated against by any program activity supported by and receiving federal aid or assistance. Thus any firm that obtains more than $2,500 of federal funds and contracts per year must adhere to this law or risk loss of the funding.

Many states encourage employers to hire the handicapped. The state government may offer a secondary injury fund to the employer, so that if a handicapped individual is injured on the job, he is paid from state funds rather than the cost being borne by the employer. However, neither the employer nor the employee can obtain this aid unless the employer is informed of the worker's epilepsy before the accident occurs.

Vocational Rehabilitation and Preparation Programs

Some epileptic individuals may be prepared for employment through involvement in special brief training programs, such as projects of the State Division of Vocational Rehabilitation services or certain Epilepsy Foundation of America sponsored projects, e.g., TAPS. A training program may convert the unemployable person to an employable one. With others, a longer placement in a more sheltered training and work situation may be necessary. This may prove to be a permanent placement.

Individuals with epilepsy who need assistance in obtaining appropriate employment may find help through the state and federal employment offices, through local employment services for the handicapped, and through the State Division of Vocational Rehabilitation (DVR).

Vocational Rehabilitation The state vocational rehabilitation agencies and their programs have been required to develop plans advancing employment services to the handicapped. Usually the eligibility age is 16 years minimum, although some programs are more liberal. Some programs work as a team with school districts and extend aid to younger adolescents.

Individuals with epilepsy who are determined by local VR counselors to have rehabilitative potential may qualify for a vocational rehabilitation program. This provides the patient assistance in medical and psychologic examinations and treatment as well as vocational evaluation, training, counseling, and assistance in job placement.

A vocational rehabilitation counselor, either as part of an epilepsy medical team or working in close association with a physician, is a valuable addition to good seizure management. The counselor is most helpful in providing the needed employment information and working to identify employability skills as well as in counseling the patient regarding other problems. A good counselor extends his services to a younger age, beginning with vocational preparatory approaches with younger children. He works with the home and the school as well as the patient so that the patient will be emotionally and academically ready to enter into a more formal vocational training experience when he reaches the age of eligibility. Some patients can succeed with just the counseling, whereas others may require involvement in a full rehabilitative program.

Individuals unable to participate in a regular vocational program because of their epilepsy or some other problem may qualify for special vocational education placement, work study programs, or a cooperative vocational rehabilitation-educational study combination within a school district. Other patients may not be able to qualify for or succeed in any competitive employment situation. They may be eligible for a sheltered workshop placement for the severely disabled through the Division of Vocational Rehabilitation. Information about sheltered, transitional, and training workshops as well as other vocational rehabilitation services can be obtained through the state or local division of vocational rehabilitation.

Epihap and Epilab Projects In some vocational rehabilitation centers, new and innovative projects aimed at helping the disabled epileptic person are being developed. These programs utilize an interdisciplinary team approach, uniting physician, psychologists, educators, counselors, and others in helping the disabled epileptic client develop a better understanding and control over his epilepsy and its consequences. Efforts are made to overcome undesirable behaviors, to improve self-concepts, to improve medical control, to regulate the patient's lifestyle, to further independent living, and to maximize the employability potential. These goals are approached through various psychosocial counseling methods, work-training experiences, formal classes, and recreational activities. Initially, a full diagnostic evaluation is completed and then the rehabilitative effort, aimed at obtaining successful employment for each client, is undertaken. Such a program is not meant to be a long-term workshop placement but rather is looked upon as an intensified short-term training approach.

When such a project is located in a major rehabilitative institute, the project may be limited in its selection criteria. People with epilepsy and additional disabilities may not qualify for the program. However, the project itself has the opportunity to share its expertise in consultation and help for other epileptic individuals in other programs. The total number of patients at the facilities, when all programs are considered, may be large enough that a self-help group may be formed from the special project and other service efforts. Thus a project intensively serving 10 to 20 people may be swelled to serve 80 to 100. This affords the project directors the opportunity to see how well their methods can be learned by fewer training counselors.

Self-Help Groups An approach used by some centers is to hold a series of structured group sessions followed by an opportunity for informal group discussions. A professional expert may be enlisted to present a review of a specific problem area related to epilepsy; e.g., legal rights, the laws, and common restrictions regarding driving, insurance, vocational rehabilitation services, scholarship and tuition assistance programs, and other agencies and resources. Also covered are the basics of the medical aspects and drug treatment of epilepsy. One-to-one counseling, group sharing experiences, vocational counseling, and referral assistance involving other agencies when needed are valuable components. Literature and films can be used to further awareness. The goals are to help the individual develop and cope with the challenges of his epilepsy. Although he may graduate from the program, he may be invited to return as part of a transitional graduate group as he passes from self-education to educating others about the management of the problems.

TAPS (Training and Placement Service) The Labor Department and the Epilepsy Foundation of America have combined to promote increased employment of epileptic individuals by providing support services and on-the-job training through a special project nicknamed TAPS. The TAPS client arrives at the potential employer's office having received individual vocational counseling in order that he may be more aware of his strengths as well as his limitations. He is referred to specific jobs that seem appropriate to his interests and capabilities. He has received special training in job-seeking techniques as well as in the acceptance and coping with his epilepsy in an employment situation.

TAPS offers the employer an appropriate candidate and backs her with on-the-job training funds to pay part of the salary during the trial period. The TAPS counselors continue ongoing contacts with the employer and the employee, offering further counseling whenever necessary. The TAPS program can offer educational services to promote understanding about epilepsy for the employer and for his other employees.

Thus the TAPS project offers the employer an appropriate referral who has already received vocational training and is backed by on-the-job training funds and client follow-up services. The client benefits from vocational counseling, job-seeking skill training, work-support groups, placement assistance, educational services, and follow-up support. An employer can help by providing the applicant a chance to work. He also can contact the program whenever he has or knows of a possible job opening. He can encourage similar participation by his business associates.

CETA (Comprehensive Employment and Training Act) Unemployed and underemployed epileptic patients may qualify for training and support as well as placement in an appropriate job through the CETA program. This program may support the patient in a job in a public or a private organization.

SOCIAL SECURITY BENEFITS

Few people with epilepsy are so handicapped that they cannot work if they are given a chance, but some individuals cannot work because their seizures are too severe or too frequent. The Social Security Administration has several programs that can provide financial assistance and, in some cases, rehabilitative training. These programs may be linked to Medicare and Medicaid programs. The local Social Security office can help eligible patients qualify for these benefits.

Supplemental Security Income (SSI)

SSI benefits, as mandated under the Social Security Act, Title XVI, offers direct cash benefits for living expenses to the blind, the aged, or other disabled patients. Individuals with severe epilepsy may qualify. Low-income families may also qualify for other services, such as Medicaid, vocational rehabilitation, various social services, or food stamps. The epileptic patient must be documented as having severely handicapping seizures. The criteria include: 1) having more than one "grand mal" or psychomotor seizure per month or more than one "petit mal" attack per week, 2) having a sufficiently low income and minimum resources, and 3) being unable to obtain any substantial gainful employment or a suitable job placement or being unable to work because of additional disabilities or drug reactions that impair his performance. These benefits have been extended to include certain disabled children.

Childhood Disability Benefits Monthly cash assistance may be made to an individual age 18 years and over who was disabled before 22 years of age. He must be so handicapped that he cannot earn more than $200 a month at best. Some disabled children already are receiving other Social Security benefits because of a parent or grandparent (see Social Security Disability Insurance). To continue these benefits, an application should be submitted on behalf of the disabled child about three months before his 18th birthday. An individual may qualify for one or the other program but not both.

Social Security benefits awarded because of a disability continue as long as the client remains too handicapped to obtain regular work. If the patient attempts to work, the benefits continue up to a nine-month period in case the patient is unable to succeed. This period need not be consecutive months. If the client succeeds, the childhood benefits may continue several months longer and then end. If he does not succeed the benefits are continued. If the individual, after a successful work period, becomes no longer employable because of the original handicap, the childhood benefits may be resumed if no more than seven years have passed. A parent caring for a disabled child may also be eligible for monthly assistance, no matter what the age of the child is. These benefits may continue even into old age, as long as the individual remains disabled and meets the eligibility requirements.

Social Security Disability Insurance

Old age insurance, under the Social Security Act, Title II, provides disability insurance to a disabled employee, his surviving spouse, or his child, provided the worker has been employed long enough or recently enough to be eligible. These benefits may be awarded to a worker who becomes disabled, or to a disabled widow or widower (occasionally a divorcee) over 50 years of age whose spouse was covered by Social Security, or for a disabled dependent over 18 years old whose handicap began before 22 years of age, whose parent (occasionally a grandparent) was covered by the Social Security Act and died, retired, or became disabled himself. The benefits are based on the earnings of the prime employee at the time of retirement, disability, or death.

The benefits will continue as long as the disabled individual remains eligible. A parent caring for an eligible disabled dependent may also be eligible to receive monthly assistance payments. The disabled beneficiary may become eligible for other services, such as Medicare and various vocational rehabilitative services.

Medicare and Medicaid

Under the Social Security Act, Title 18 and 19, certain cash assistance may be awarded in payment for medical and other services that an epileptic patient needs. Medicare is based on age, on catastrophic illness, or on severe disability, whereas Medicaid is based on need.

Medicare If an epileptic patient qualifies under the disability insurance program, he may be eligible to receive assistance to help pay for physician, clinic, and hospital fees, hospitalization and post-hospitalization care costs, medical and social services and supplies (except drugs), and other health service expenses. The beneficiary must pay a portion of the cost for each service. If the patient is under 65 years of age, he may have to be on the Social Security Disability Payment program for 24 consecutive months before he becomes eligible for Medicare.

Medicaid Low-income epileptic patients may be eligible for county and state aid through federal matching assistance. This may help in the payment of hospital and clinic fees, physician costs, laboratory charges, transportation expenses, and some nursing aid. SSI benefits may help qualify the patients for these services.

The eligibility qualifications and benefits of these Social Security services, like other governmental assistance programs, are under constant revision. If the epileptic patient thinks she may be eligible for a certain program, it is wise to contact the agency involved, to review the specific eligibility requirements, and to pursue the benefits if she seems to qualify.

RESOURCES FOR HELP

The family and the individual with epilepsy are constantly bombarded with a volley of restrictions and a mountain of expenses. Many times the family is overwhelmed and does not know where to search for help. There are numerous resources available, as is evident in the preceding discussion on employment and social security. However, the physician and the family may not be aware of the existence of these resources.

Medical Help

Medical resources may be found by contacting medical centers and clinics, the local and state department of health, the community mental health facilities, or a medical school teaching hospital, if a local physician is not available. For more complicated cases, an interdisciplinary team, including a nurse specialist, a psychologist, an educator, a social worker, a vocational rehabilitation counselor, an early childhood developmental specialist, a speech and language therapist, a special educator, a mental health counselor, and a person able to assist in outreach programs in awareness and service development in local communities, is desirable in addition to a physician who is interested, available, knowledgeable, and active in trying to help the epileptic patient. This would be the ideal approach both for direct care and for aiding other physicians and services working with the epileptic individual. Such programs are seldom available. The University Affiliated Programs (UAP, UAC, or UAF) and the Comprehensive Epilepsy Centers scattered across the nation come closest to meeting these ideal approaches.

The medical costs and the expenses in dealing with related problems can be overwhelming. Medical cost assistance for low-income families, severely disabled individuals, or those qualifying through the various social security benefits for the disabled, may be obtained. Low-income groups may qualify for medical care through the various state programs, such as the Crippled Children's Services, the Departments of Health and Welfare, the Division of Vocational Rehabilitation, the Maternal and Infant or Child Health programs, various social securities programs, or other local projects. These services vary from state to state, as do the eligibility criteria.

Health services, especially in low-income areas, may be provided through the Maternal and Child Health services. Often these cover the care of epilepsy. In many states, epilepsy care is provided to low-income families through the Crippled Children's Services. These services include diagnostic and management services, as well as payment for medicines, needed appliances, and necessary hospitalizations. Sometimes transportation to and from the clinical facilities is arranged. The Department of Welfare or the Red Cross also may be contacted for transportation assistance. Assistance in buying medicines may be obtained for some through the Department of Welfare or through various Medicare or Medicaid programs. For those who do not qualify for these governmental services or for the medical benefits offered by various unions and industrial corporations, the Epilepsy Foundation of America does provide a discount drug service for the needed anticonvulsants.

Vital services in dentistry and nursing care also may be available to epileptic patients. Dental care may be obtained through the local or state departments of health or the state schools of dentistry, if a private dentist is not available. Nursing assistance and instruction may be obtained through the local and state public health nurses, the Crippled Children's services, or the Visiting Nurses Association.

Individuals whose epilepsy originated in childhood, and in whom the seizures have become a chronic, significantly disabling problem, may qualify for specialized services through the state Developmental Disabilities programs, whenever such services are available. These services may include help in caring for the patient, group homes, special therapeutic efforts, special projects, and various rehabilitative services. Although the major developmental disabilities include mental retardation, cerebral palsy, epilepsy, autism, and to some degree specific learning disabilities, some states expand their efforts to include other handicaps. The type of services and projects often reflect the pressures and desires of various active advocacy organizations in the state. The most active groups influence the most active projects. Unless the state's advocate for epilepsy is especially active, the programs tend to be oriented toward some of the other developmental disabilities, such as mental retardation.

The University Affiliated Programs The UAF (alias UAC or UAP Programs) present as a multidisciplinary approach to the diagnosis, remediation, research, and training in improving the care of the developmentally disabled person. It is an independent program but it is affiliated with a university. This program can potentially offer much toward helping in awareness, care, and training in improved total management of the consequences of epilepsy for students from various disciplines. Often the efforts tend to become oriented toward services versus research, education versus medicine, or retardation versus epilepsy and other problems. The most successful programs are those that have retained their balance.

Education

Educational help and referral to appropriate services can be obtained by contacting the departments of education and special education in the city, county, or state school system or the educational divisions of colleges and universities. Other resources for help include the Crippled Children's Services, community mental health centers, state departments of health or mental health, or a university affiliated program.

Early Infancy or Childhood Stimulation Programs In some states, programs are being developed through community mental health centers or the Easter Seal centers to provide early intervention and stimulation for neonates, infants, and often toddlers who have been identified as having a known or suspected developmental delay or disability. These programs offer a variety of services, both diagnostic and remediative, such as training in movement and coordination, in speech and language development, in social interactions, in self-help skills, in physical therapy, and in general development. They not only serve the patient directly but also work with the parent both at the center and in the patient's home, training the parents in awareness and various approaches so that they may be involved in stimulating and encouraging proper development.

Head Start A child of 3 to 6 years of age from a low-income family may be able to qualify for the Head Start program or for a related project. A certain percentage of children in these programs must have a handicap, such as epilepsy. These programs may be a part of a developmental continuity of services under a variety of nicknames, such as Follow-Through, PUSH, etc. The Head Start project offers a variety of services, including educational and social services, and psychological, nursing, medical, dental, and nutritional help. For the epileptic child the services might aid with diagnosis, medical care, therapy, transportation, special equipment or materials, adapting physical facilities to the child's needs, or in observing the child and training the parents about epilepsy.

Right to an Education As discussed in the previous chapter on learning, every child, no matter what his handicap, has the right to an appropriate educational experience through the public school system. Under the Education for All Handicapped Children Act (PL 94-142 or 1975), all children between ages 3 and 21 who have been shown to require some type of specialized educational service must receive it. By law, the schools must directly or indirectly provide the services to all eligible children, both the unserved and the underserved. This is a federally funded effort. Any state or local school system that does not comply with the mandate is in danger of losing its federal funds.

This effort is an outgrowth of the Vocational Rehabilitation Act of 1973. It applies to ages 3 to 18 as of September 1978 and is extended to age 21 by September 1980, unless it is inconsistent with an existing state law, practice, or court decree. Yet the parents have the right to persist and to pursue the mandated programs, utilizing professional assistance, advocacy groups, and medical support, until they obtain what is needed and what by right should be available. However, it is far better to try to work out a mutually satisfactory program with the school rather than to become involved in angry confrontations that include legal help; the latter may win a battle of temporary appropriate placement, but lose an overall war by stigmatizing the child and his siblings for the remainder of their school careers.

Emotional Problems

Psychological services, counseling, and psychiatric help with emotional problems and behavioral difficulties can be obtained through community mental health centers, local and state mental health organizations, the state department or division of mental health, the departments of behavioral medicine or psychiatry in medical centers, departments of psychology at various colleges, vocational rehabilitation services, or sometimes an interested, trained, and concerned minister. Community mental health centers are developed to provide 24-hour services to patients with all types of emotional problems. Because of the common association of childhood problems with school and developmental difficulties, many organizations have also become quite active in these areas. If the mental health center or other resources are able to develop understanding and expertise in handling the emotional problems of epilepsy, they can be very valuable resources. Part of good management of epilepsy and its consequences involves some degree of emotional counseling aimed at both the patient and his family.

Housing

Low-income families who have problems with housing may obtain assistance from the local department of public welfare. This department, like the public health department and various other social agencies, may be able to help in locating extended care and residential care facilities for epileptic individuals.

The resources that have been discussed above are summarized in Table 14.1.

Table 14.1 Resources for possible individual benefits

Type of Benefit	Eligibility	Agency
Supplemental Security Income (SSI)	Low income Disabled	Social Security
Disability insurance	Eligible worker, his spouse or child, disabled	Social Security
Medicare	Eligible for disability insurance for 24 months	Social Security Designated agencies
Medicaid	Low income SSI Eligible	Public Welfare Public Health
Maternal and Child Health Services	Low-income area	State and local projects
Crippled Children's Services	Low income Defined handicap	Local project State agency
Social services, such as day care, case management, homemaker services, counseling	SSI eligible Low income	State or county social service agencies; other agencies
Comprehensive epilepsy centers; other similar projects	Research grants Project fundings	Medical schools
University affiliated centers	Project fundings Research grants	Universities
Community mental health centers	Need: Adjustable fees	Local mental health agency
Early childhood stimulation projects	Child of 0 to 3-5 years with known or suspected risk of development	Local mental health center; Easter Seals Program
Head Start	Age 3 to 6 years, low-income family, 10% handicapped children	Local school administration of federal grant
Education for All Handicapped	Age 3 to 21 years, proven disability and specialized educational needs	Local school district; State Department of Education

Table 14.1 — *continued*

Type of Benefit	Eligibility	Agency
Special vocational education, work study or vocational-education cooperative program	Adult or child unable to succeed in regular vocational program due to handicap	Local school district
Job development and placement services	Epileptic persons Desire to work	Local employment office
Sheltered workshops	Epileptic persons Unable to work	Non-profit workshops State Vocational Rehabilitation agency
Comprehensive job training and support services (CETA)	Unemployed and underemployed epileptics	Local CETA sponsor or sub-grantee
Comprehensive vocational rehabilitation services	Potentially employable epileptic persons	Local and state vocational rehabilitation offices
Removal of architectural barriers	All handicapped individuals	Employer, local or regional HEW office, Officer of Compliance Board, in Washington
Specialized habilitation services	Childhood onset, Chronic disabling epilepsy	Developmental disability programs
Legal services in civil matters	Low income (fees are adjustable)	Local legal services and Legal Aid offices
Low-cost housing	Low income area	Local housing agency
Comprehensive medical and rehabilitative services	Veterans	Veterans hospital

ADVOCACY AND THE LAW

Under the Vocational Rehabilitation Act of 1973, the amendment of 1974, and the Rights of the Handicapped to an Appropriate Education Act of 1975, the epileptic individual and his family have the right to expect certain services. The individual is protected against any discrimination in employment. He is given the right to expect programs developed to offer him an employment opportunity. He can expect that any architectural barriers that inhibit him because of his handicap be removed. Yet these laws were passed prior to the passage of an effective method of enforcement. This required the development of an agency to monitor, protect, and stimulate advocacy on behalf of the disabled. The state advocacy programs tend to function as agencies of information and referral. Often the client who has a problem is referred to a lawyer for help in resolving potential legal barriers toward gaining the desired services.

For example, if an employee is dismissed because of his epilepsy, he may seek legal help to get his job back. A similar situation may exist if the applicant is refused a job or entry into a college because of his epilepsy. A lawsuit, based on the laws presently effective, may be successfully won unless the employer can demonstrate that the handicap directly affects the worker's ability to perform a job successfully. Similarly, a child who is refused needed and mandated services by a school may take that school to court.

The state advocacy council, along with local organizations fighting for the rights of the handicapped individual and the lawyers involved in the cases, must keep abreast of the pertinent statutes, laws, and regulations, including those pertaining to the Vocational Rehabilitation and Social Security Acts as well as the Right to Education Acts. They must be aware of court decisions in similar cases elsewhere. The Epilepsy Foundation of America offers a text, *The Legal Rights of Persons with Epilepsy,* that gives a state-by-state review of laws specifically affecting epileptic citizens. The EFA also has a growing legal division that may be able to help with significant problems. The local advocacy group for epilepsy, working with advocacy groups for other disabilities, must continually monitor the efforts of the state programs.

Whenever a patient or a family feel that their rights have been denied, they may either seek local counsel or contact their state advocacy representative for assistance. Legal help may also be obtained from the American Civil Liberties Union, local offices of Legal Aid, the Public Defender, or a university school of law if the client cannot afford a personal lawyer. The advocacy agency should monitor all grievances and refer the individual to a lawyer versed in the specific area of need. It may have to supply him with needed case examples. The counsel should be sure that a true grievance exists; if not, it should discuss this with the complaining party. The counsel should monitor the case to completion. It should gather data to be given to state officials and agencies so that better services can be developed.

The lawyer's primary duty is to advise and counsel, not to bring lawsuits. He should give his opinions and suggestions about what may be the best overall approach to resolving the problem. If needed, then he may go with the family and the patient to the school or employer to speak for the rights of his client. If all else fails, then he may need to turn to a lawsuit through the courts.

CONCLUSION

The restrictions placed by a rejecting society often become more handicapping than the seizures themselves. However, there are resources and rights that can help overcome these restrictions. Purely medically-oriented management may help control the seizures but it may not help the patient. Through either lack of awareness or lack of interest, a medical team may fail to acquaint the patient with the restrictions he faces.

REFERENCES AND SUGGESTED READING

General

Aird, R. B., and D. M. Woodbury. 1974. The Management of Epilepsy. Charles C Thomas, Springfield, Ill. 448 pp.
Bagley, C. 1972. Social prejudice and the adjustment of people with epilepsy. Epilepsia 13:33-45.
Boshes, L. D., and H. W. Kienst. 1972. Community aspects of epilepsy — a modern reappraisal. Epilepsia 13:31-32.
Caveness, W. F., H. H. Merritt, and G. H. Gallup, Jr. 1974. A survey of public attitudes toward epilepsy in 1974 with an indication of trends over the past twenty-five years. Epilepsia 15:523-536.
(The) Commission for the Control of Epilepsy and Its Consequences. 1977-78. Plan for Nationwide Action on Epilepsy. United States Printing Office. DHEW Pub. No. (NIH) 78-276. 4 Vol.
Epilepsy Foundation of America. 1975. Basic Statistics on the Epilepsies. F. A. Davis Co., Philadelphia, p. 155.
Livingston, S. 1972. Comprehensive Management of Epilepsy in Infancy, Childhood and Adolescence. Charles C Thomas, Springfield, Ill. 657 pp.
Sands, H., and F. C. Minters. 1977. The Epilepsy Fact Book. F. A. Davis Co., Philadelphia. 116 pp.
Solomon, G. E., and F. Plum. 1976. Clinical Management of Seizures. W. B. Saunders Company, Philadelphia. 152 pp.

Driving

Van der Lugt, P. J. M. 1975. Is an application form useful to select patients who may drive? Epilepsia 16:743-746.
Van der Lugt, P. J. M. 1975. Traffic accidents caused by epilepsy. Epilepsia 16: 747-752.

Education

Scheiber, B. (ed.) 1977. You have new rights — Use them! In: Report from Closer Look, National Information Center for the Handicapped, Special Issue, Fall, 1977. P. O. Box 1492, Washington, D. C. 20013.

Employment

Epilepsy Foundation of America. Training and Placement Services, Suite 406, 1928 L Street, N.W., Washington, D.C. 20036.
National Association of Epilepsy Executives, 4438 South 365th Street, Arlington, Virginia 22206.
Perlman, L. G., and L. A. Studler. 1976. The epileptic citizen, an employment perspective. J. Rehab. March-April 1976, pp. 36-40.
Rodin, E., P. Rennick, R. Dennerll, and Y. Lin. 1972. Vocational and educational problems of epileptic patients. Epilepsia 13:149-160.

Wright, G. N. 1975. Epilepsy Rehabilitation. Little, Brown & Company, Boston. 275 pp.

Sports

AMA Committee on Exercise and Physical Fitness. 1968. Convulsive disorders and participation in sports and physical education. JAMA 206:1291.

Committee on Children with Handicaps. 1968. The epileptic child and competitive school activities. Pediatrics 42:700.

15
THE FUTURE

Roughly one in every one hundred people is under active care for seizures. Medical advances that save lives or prolong life, such as the newborn high-risk programs, modern intensive care units, and new breakthroughs in medical care, as well as increasing public awareness of, acceptance of, and hope for better seizure control may tend to increase the percentage of individuals with epilepsy.

DIAGNOSIS

Only about 80% to 90% of people with seizures are confirmed as epileptic by the EEG. Over-reliance on the EEG and under-reliance on a good clinical history and observation may lead to errors in diagnosis, both in missing handicapping seizures and in over-diagnosing epilepsy, with the result that the individual suffers unjustifiably.

RESPONSE TO MEDICATIONS

About half of seizure patients can achieve quick, total control over their attacks with appropriate medical care. An additional third usually achieve good control with an infrequent breakthrough attack. A small group of epileptic patients may be improved but never seem to achieve satisfactory control despite intensive and excellent medical efforts. It is this latter group that is anxiously awaiting new research breakthroughs.

The best outlook exists when the patient has no other abnormalities, handicaps, or indications of accompanying brain damage. He may only have one or at most two generalized motor seizures. The initial EEG may be normal or it soon becomes relatively normal. Seizures that become controlled quickly with only one or two drugs often have a good outlook.

Seizures of a mixed type, seizures of very early onset, or distinctly focal seizures that occur frequently have a more guarded outlook. The seizures may eventually be controlled, but the patient commonly is left with other handicaps. The outlook for eventual good control is reduced if the attacks recur frequently, begin at an early age, are very focal, or are not controlled after a prolonged period of intensive and appropriate anticonvulsant efforts.

Some types of seizures are easier to control than others. Simple generalized tonic-clonic motor attacks, simple absence seizures, and simple focal attacks are often fairly easily controlled. Psychomotor seizures may be more difficult to control. Complicated seizure types, such as complex focal seizures, or, even more so, atypical absence seizures and the related myoclonic and akinetic attacks, as well as mixed seizure patterns and seizures following obvious brain damage, often prove difficult to control.

The chances for total seizure control are best with simple absence attacks and simple febrile seizures. Often the patient seems to outgrow the tendency toward these seizures. The expectation for total control is not as high with generalized tonic-clonic motor attacks, simple focal seizures, and psychomotor seizures. If the attacks occur more often than once a year, the outlook for total control is not good. Atypical absence attacks, akinetic attacks, and minor myoclonic attacks are often very difficult to totally control. Infantile myoclonic spasms may disappear with age but the patient often is left severely handicapped by slowed mental development; he may also have multiple residual seizures or generalized motor attacks, although not infrequently he may outgrow any seizure tendency and be able to discontinue his medicine.

The age of the patient is significant. The tendency toward seizures and the appearance and types of seizures vary with age. In the neonate, fragmentary seizures are most common. The infant is apt to present with myoclonic or generalized motor attacks. The child of 5 to 7 years of age seems especially prone to absence attacks. Psychomotor seizures become prominent, or at least are more easily recognized, by adolescence to early adulthood. Seizures that begin in early childhood, before age 4, may be rather easily controlled. The exception seems to be seizures that begin in early infancy. However, this control may be temporary. There is a tendency for these seizures to recur in adolescence or in the preadolescent years between 9 to 15 years of age. This period of recurrence may last for 4 to 7 years, then cease.

The use of medication plays an important role in the outlook. The chances for preventing the recurrence of a seizure are quite high if the patient is placed on anticonvulsant medicine after the first seizure. Some physicians prefer to wait until a second seizure occurs before beginning the anticonvulsant drug. The chances are fairly good that a second seizure will occur. However, some patients may never have a second attack. A drug that is properly used and monitored by several blood level measurements will probably be effective within the first six months of therapy. If no effect is seen by then, the medication is probably not going to work and should be slowly discontinued.

The length of time that the patient remains on a medication while his seizures remain controlled is controversial. The estimates range from 2 to 5 completely seizure-free years before gradual stopping of the medicine. The chances of recurrence after 3 or 4 years of total control is rather low. Usually the recurrence will happen while the drug is being tapered off in the first few months after stopping the medicine. If a recurrence has not occurred within the first few years, it probably will not happen in the future. The one exception is the tendency for early childhood seizures to recur in early adolescence.

OVERALL OUTLOOK

The risks and chances for success that may be quoted to the patient or family about a desired response to medicines or the chance for good seizure control, like the risk of recurrence after slowly discontinuing the medicine, are still vague estimates. The outlook for a successful life is not measured by just control versus non-control of seizures; it depends on the patient's ability to overcome the emotional turmoils, behavioral reactions, earning difficulties, and social attitudes and restrictions that persist as the major handicap long after the last pill has been stopped and the last attack has occurred. The physician who treats only seizures may have controlled the convulsions but failed the patient; the physician who treats the epileptic patient, his seizures, and the consequences of his epilepsy is truly successful, since he helps the whole patient.

REFERENCES AND SUGGESTED READING

Epilepsy Foundation of America. 1975. Basic Statistics on the Epilepsies. F. A. Davis Co., Philadelphia. 155 pp.

Holowach, J., D. L. Thurston, and J. O'Leary. 1969. Prognosis in childhood epilepsy: Follow-up of 148 cases in which therapy has been suspended after prolonged anticonvulsant control. New Engl. J. Med. 286:169–174.

Iuul-Jensen, P. 1974. Social prognosis. In: O. Magnus and A. M. Lorentz de Haas (eds.), The Epilepsies, Vol. 15. P. J. Vincken and G. W. Bruyn (eds.), Handbook of Clinical Neurology, Chapter 41, pp. 800–814. Elsevier-North Holland Publishing Company, New York.

Kiorboe, E. 1974. Medical prognosis of epilepsy. In: O. Magnus and A. M. Lorentz de Haas (eds.), The Epilepsies, Vol. 15. P. J. Vincken and G. W. Bruyn (eds.), Handbook of Clinical Neurology, Chapter 40, pp. 783–799. Elsevier-North Holland Publishing Company, New York.

Sands, H., and F. C. Minters. 1977. The Epilepsy Fact Book. F. A. Davis Co., Philadelphia. 116 pp.

Appendix
RESOURCES FOR FURTHER INFORMATION AND HELP

RESOURCES FOR FURTHER INFORMATION AND HELP

General Summary of Facts, Programs, Needs, and Recommendations

Plan for Nationwide Action on Epilepsy, reported by the Commission for the Control of Epilepsy and Its Consequences. 4 Volumes. DHEW Publication No. (NIH) 78-276. The Office of Scientific and Health Reports. Room 8408, Building 31. NINICDS-NIH, Bethesda, Md. 20014, 1978.

Basic Statistics on the Epilepsies. Prepared by the Epilepsy Foundation of America. F. A. Davis Co., Philadelphia. 1975. 155 pp.

Resources for Information, Assistance, Materials, Films, etc.

Epilepsy Foundation of America (EFA). 1828 L Street, N.W., Suite 406, Washington, D. C. 20036

Closer Look. The National Information Center for the Handicapped, Box 1492, Washington, D.C. 20013

Drug Company Sources of Films and Teaching Materials

Ayerst Medical Information Services. Audiovisual Library of Ayerst Laboratories, 685 Third Avenue, New York, N.Y. 10017

Geigy Pharmaceutical Company, Division of CIBA-GEIGY Corporation, Ardsley, N.Y. 10502

Hoffman La Roche, Inc. Nutley, N.J. 07110

Parke Davis and Company, P.O. Box 118A, Dept. 5721, Detroit, Mich. 48232

Directories of Clinical Services

A National Director of Clinical Facilities for the Treatment and Diagnosis of Persons with Epilepsy. *See* Epilepsy Foundation of America.

Team Clinical Programs

Comprehensive Epilepsy Programs associated with: Medical College of Georgia (Augusta, Georgia), University of Minnesota (Minneapolis or Rochester), Epilepsy Center of Oregon, University of Oregon (Portland), University of Virginia (Charlottesville), University of Washington Epilepsy Center (Seattle), Epilepsy Center of Michigan (Lafayette), Northern New Jersey Neurological Consultation Service (Affiliated with Columbia University)

University Affiliated Programs, Suite 406, 2033 M Street, N.W., Washington, D.C. 20036

Newspaper on Epilepsy

The National Spokesman (the official newsletter of the Epilepsy Foundation of America) and chapter newsletters, *see* Epilepsy Foundation of America.

Reading Materials to Begin Learning

General — For Anyone

The Epilepsy Fact Book (soft cover) by H. Sands and F. C. Minters. F. A. Davis Co., Philadelphia. 1977. (116 pp.)

The Child with Convulsions: A Guide for Parents, Teachers, Counselors, and Medical Personnel, by H. W. Baird. Grune & Stratton, New York. 1972. (144 pp.)

Epilepsy (soft cover), by Alvin and V. B. Silverstein. J. B. Lippincott Company, Philadelphia. 1975. (64 pp.)

Numerous pamphlets, brochures and bulletins from the Epilepsy Foundation of America, on general and individual discipline topics.

Pamphlet listing books on the epilepsies for the lay and professional reader, subdivided into (a) patient or parent, (b) social worker, educator, vocational rehabilitation counselor, (c) student, (d) physician or nurse, can be obtained from the Epilepsy Foundation of America.

Family

Seizures, Epilepsy, and Your Child, by J. C. Lagos. Harper and Row Publishers, New York. 1974. (238 pp.)

Gripping Tales or Living with Seizures (soft cover), a booklet by a class of children with epilepsy. The Wisconsin Epilepsy Association, 1245 East Washington Ave., Madison, Wisconsin 53703

Handbooks for Patients, for Parents (soft cover), each by H. S. Barrows and E. S. Goldensohn. Distributed by Ayerst Laboratories.

Teachers and School Nurse

Epilepsy School Alert Packet, obtainable from the Epilepsy Foundation of America.

Comprehensive Management of Epilepsy in Infancy, Childhood, and Adolescence, by S. Livingston. Charles C Thomas Publishing Company, Springfield, Ill. 1972. (657 pp.)

The Social Psychology of the Epileptic Child, by C. Bagley. University of Miami Publishers, Coral Gables, Florida. 1971. (307 pp.)

The Mid-Career Epileptic. Problems of the Onset of Epilepsy in Adulthood, by S. T. Barry. Epilepsy Society of Massachusetts, Boston, Mass. 1971. (21 pp.)

The Rehabilitation of the Young Epileptic, by G. J. Golden. D.C. Health Publishers, Boston, Mass. 1971. (130 pp.)

Medical Personnel

Clinical Management of Seizures, a Guide for the Physician (soft cover), by G. E. Solomon and F. Plum. W. B. Saunders Company, Philadelphia. 1976. (152 pp.)

Seizures and Other Paroxysmal Disorders in Infants and Children, by M. R. Gomez and D. W. Klass. Current Problems in Pediatrics, Vol. 2, No. 6 & 7. Year Book Medical Publishers, Inc., Chicago. 1972. (75 pp.)

The Management of Epilepsy, by R. B. Aird and D. M. Woodbury. Charles C Thomas Publishing Company, Springfield, Ill. 1974. (448 pp.)

Legal Information

Legal Rights of Persons with Epilepsies, published by the Epilepsy Foundation of America.

Epilepsy and the Law (Ed. 2), by R. L. Barrow and H. D. Fabing. Hoeber Medical Division of Harper and Row Publishers, New York. 1966. (174 pp.)

Employment Services and Information

Training and Placement Services (TAPS): Contact Project Director at the Epilepsy Foundation of America.

National Association of Epilepsy Executives, 4438 South 36th Street, Arlington, Virginia 22206

Films about Epilepsy (by the Epilepsy Foundation of America unless indicated otherwise)

General Public

Epilepsy: Don't Look Away

Doctors Talk About Epilepsy

Not Without Hope (M. Faber Productions, 6412 Desert Cove, Scottsdale, Arizona 85254)

Children

Benjamin, a cartoon (Epilepsy Society of Massachusetts, 3 Arlington Street, Boston, Massachusetts 02116)

Because You Are My Friend

Teachers

Epilepsy: For Those Who Teach

Images of Epilepsy (Colorado Epilepsy Association, 1835 Gaylord St., Denver, Colorado 80206)

Convulsions (Lawren Productions Inc., P.O. Box 1542, Burlington, Calif. 94010)

Counselors, Vocational Rehabilitation Counselors

New Day for Epileptics (National Educational Television, 10 Columbus Circle, New York, N.Y. 10019)

Epilepsy: Pass the Word

Epilepsy: The Invisible Wound (Colorado Epilepsy Association, 1835 Gaylord St., Denver, Colorado 80206)

Branded Imperfect (National Archives Trust Fund, National Audio Visual Center, Attn: Reference Section, GSA, Washington, D.C. 20409)

Nurses

Nurses Talk About Epilepsy

Modern Concepts of Epilepsy (Ayerst Laboratories, Cat. #10561)

Grand Mal Epilepsy, Diagnosis and Management (Ayerst Laboratories, Cat. #10531)

Physicians and Nurses

Diagnosis and Medical Management of Epileptic Seizures (Ayerst Laboratories, Cat. #10620)

The Absence Seizure (AVELINE, Educational Materials Project, Association of American Medical Colleges. One Dupont Circle, N.W., Washington, D.C. 20036)

Public Service Personnel

Epilepsy: For Those Who Help

Auditory Tape Cassettes

Understanding and Living with Epilepsy (Designed for counselors and the family of the child with epilepsy, by the Epilepsy Foundation of America.)

Slide-Audiocassette Learning Systems

Seizure Disorders: Diagnosis and Clinical Management (Developed by the Health Learning Systems, Inc., as sponsored by the Epilepsy Foundation of America, distributed by Parke Davis and Company, P.O. Box 118A, Dept. 5721, Detroit, Michigan 48232.)

Medical Alert Bracelets, Necklaces, Discs, Tags

Medic Alert Foundation, Box 1009, Turlock, California 95380

National Identification Company, Inc., 3955 Oneida St., Denver, Colorado 80207

Emergency Medical Identification. American Medical Association, 535 North Dearborn Street, Chicago, Illinois 60610 (for emergency identification cards)
Local chapters
Medi-Check International Foundation, Inc., 2640 Golf Road, Glenview, Illinois 60025

The amount of materials, films, brochures, tapes, and other aids for those working in the field of epilepsy and for those in need of help in understanding epilepsy and its consequences is growing more rapidly than lists can be published. At present, the Epilepsy Foundation of America has become a reference center for such materials. It is always wise to contact either the national center or a local state office to obtain additional resources, references, and aids.

Index

Abdominal epilepsy, 61
Absence seizure, *see also* Atypical absence seizure
  brainwave pattern, 75-76
  characteristics, 26-27
  duration, 62
  inheritance and, 36
  prognosis, 224
  specific medicines for, 104, 114
Achievement tests, 86-87
ACTA scan, 80
Activity, restrictions on, 202
Acupuncture, 153
Advocacy programs, 219-220
Affect disturbance, 24, 31
Age of onset, 40-41
  associated emotional problems, 157-158
  prognosis and, 224
Agranulocytosis, 128
Air studies, 82-83, 85
Akinetic drop seizure, 17, 27-28
  causes, 37
  prognosis, 224
  specific medicines for, 104, 114
Alcohol, seizures and, 135-136
Allergy, 108, 109, 125-129
Ammonium chloride, 139
Anaphylactic reaction, acute, 126
Anemia, 128
  in offspring, 132
Angiography, 81-82, 85
Anticonvulsants, 96, *see also* Drug management
  serum levels, monitoring of, 110-111
  side effects, 121-134
  toxicity rating, 104
  types of, 104-105
Arizona Test of Articulation Proficiency, 85
Astatic drop seizure, 27-28
Asymmetry, of brainwave pattern, 75, 78
Asynchrony, 75
Athetosis, 64
Atonic drop seizure, 27-28
Atypical absence seizure
  causes, 37

  prognosis, 224
  retardation risk, 194
  specific medicines for, 104, 114
Auditory Discrimination Test, 85
Aura, 9-12, 14, 20
Autism, 194
Automatism, 12, 22, 23
  with absence seizure, 27

Babinski sign, 53
Barbiturates, 96, 99, 104, *see also* specific compound
  allergic reactions to, 127
  effect on concentration, 130
  interaction with other drugs, 115
  laboratory tests during use of, 109
  teratogenic effects, 132
  withdrawal, 119
Bayley Infant Maturation Scales, 84
Beery-Buktenica Developmental Test of Visual Motor Integration, 87
Behavioral consequences
  in children, 158-160
  of epilepsy, 24, 157-184
  unhealthy attitudes, 160
  history, 47
  seizure mimics and, 58-60
  seizure types and, 164-165
Behavioral management, 145-150
Behavioral tests, 83-90
Behavior modification, 148-149
Benadryl, 129
Bender Gestalt Test, 87
Benign paroxysmal torticollis, 63
Benign paroxysmal vertigo, 61, 63
Berea Gestalt Test, 87
Biofeedback, 149-150
Birthmarks, 52
Benzodiazepines, 105
Blacky Picture Test, 88
Blood
  allergic reactions and, 128-129
  excess alkalinity, management, 100
Blood count, complete, 69-70, 109-110
Blood pressure
  anticonvulsant dosage and, 98

Blood pressure — *continued*
  during acute seizure, 49
  high, cause of seizure, 99
Blood sugar level, seizure and, 39, 70, 94-95, 100, 136
Boredom, 147
Brain
  abnormal EEG, 74-78
  cellular organization, 14
  diagnostic procedures involving, 71-83
  during seizure, 13-15
  effects of early damage, 190-191
  functional areas, 10-12
  lateralization of function, 190
  motor strip, 20, 21
  nerve cell death, 195
  sensory area, 20, 21
Brain edema, management, 101
Brain stimulators, 153
Brainwave test, *see* Electroencephalogram
Breath-holding, 62
Burst-suppression pattern, 76

Cataplexy, 60
Cattell Infant Intelligence Scale, 86
Celontin, 105, 106, 112, 114-117
  allergic reactions to, 127
  idiosyncratic reactions to, 131
  interaction with other drugs, 115
CETA, *see* Comprehensive Employment and Training Act
Childhood disability benefits, 213
Children's Apperception Test, 88
Chloral hydrate, 96, 97, 99
Chlorpromazine, 100
Chorea, 59, 64
Classification of seizure disorders, 17-31
Clonazepam, 96
Clonipin, 105, 106, 113-116, 122
  allergic reactions to, 127
  idiosyncratic reactions to, 131
  interaction with other drugs, 115
  laboratory tests during use of, 109
Cognitive disturbance, 24, 31, 88
Commission for Control of Epilepsy and Its Consequences, 1, 6-7

Comprehensive Employment and Training Act, 212, 219
Comprehensive Epilepsy Center, 215
Computerized tomography scan, 80, 84
Consciousness
  loss of, causes, 62
  loss of, as single symptom, 24
  state of, after acute seizure, 49
Constipation, 139
Counseling, 144, 176-177, 211
Crisis intervention, 145
CT scan, *see* Computerized tomography scan
Cylert, 161

Dating, 204
Decadron, 101
Decerebrate posture, 51
Decorticate posture, 51
Delta abnormality, 74, 77, 78
Demyelination, 71
Denver Developmental Screening Test, 84
Depression, 130
Detroit Test of Learning Abilities, 87
Developmental disabilities, identification, 46-47
Developmental tests, 84
Dexedrine, 161
Diagnosis
  basic tests, 69
  errors in, 223
  hospitalization and, 67-68
  laboratory studies for, 67-91
  non-invasive studies, 84
  supplemental testing, 83-90
Diamox, 39, 105, 106, 114, 115, 117, 139
  allergic reactions to, 127
  interaction with other drugs, 115
Dilantin, 96-99, 104, 106, 112-116, 192
  allergic reactions to, 127
  cosmetic effects of, 131
  idiosyncratic reactions to, 130, 131
  intelligence deterioration and, 195
  interaction with other drugs, 115, 124
  intoxication, 122, 123

laboratory tests during use of, 109
learning and, 130
teratogenic effects, 132
toxicity, 104, 105
withdrawal, 119
Driving restrictions, 203
Drug, non-anticonvulsant, seizures and, 135-136
Drug fever, 126
Drug history, 45-46
Drug interactions, 115, 124
Drug intoxication, 121-125
Drug management, see also Allergy; Anticonvulsants; Idiosyncrasy; Intoxication; Malformation
  after acute seizure, 96-102
  beginning stage, 105-108
  check-up schedule, 109-111
  dosage and form, 46, 106
  drug combination, 113-116
  frequency and time, 106-107
  during hospitalization for surgery, 112
  medication change, 113
  missed medication and, 112
  model for, 223-225
  ongoing, 103-120
  patient responsibility for, 163-164
  seizures versus intoxication, 124-125
  stages of, 103
  stomach upsets and, 111-112
  under medication, 125
  withdrawal, 116-119
Durrell Analysis of Reading Difficulty, 86
Dysrhythmia, 74-76, 78
Dystonia, 64

Echoencephalogram, 79, 84
Education, see also School
  programs in, 216-217
  right to, 196-199, 217
EEG, see Electroencephalogram
Electroencephalogram, 57, 63, 104, 118
  abnormal, 74-77, 78
  flat, 74
  normal, 74
  procedure, 71-77, 84

  timing of, 73-74
  value of, 72-73
EMI scan, 80
Emotional disturbances
  aid for, 217
  of epilepsy, 24, 157-184
  seizure mimics and, 58-60
  treatment, 170-172
  types of, 157
Emotional stability, testing of, 88-89
Employment
  problems of, 204-212
  services available, 209-212, 219
Epihap and Epilab projects, 210-211
Epilepsia partialis continuans, 94
Epileptic cry, 25
Epilepsy, see also Seizure
  associated problems, 2-6
  cost, 4
  governmental programs and, 1, 209-221
  incidence, 3-4
  life expectancy, 5
  as social stigma, 3
Erythrocyte sedimentation count, 69-70
Ether, 96, 97, 99
Examination, 45-46
  after acute seizure, 48-49
  goals of, 47-48
  neurologic, 53-55
  procedure, 50-55
Eye disorders, 63

Fainting, 62
Family, reactions of, 172-177
Febrile seizure
  age of onset, 40, 41
  cause, 39
  heritability, 36
  prognosis, 224
Fever
  after seizure, 95, 100
  seizure and, 38, 41, 53
Financial aid, 212-219
Flashing light, 73, 75, 76
Flexion spasms, 29
Fluid intake, seizures and, 139
Fluid maintenance, 100

Focal motor status, 94
Focal seizure, 18-25
  age of onset, 40, 41
  causes, 38
  of childhood, 24-25
  complicated, 19, 22-24
  definition, 14
  examination, 55
  laboratory diagnosis, 68
  mimicking conditions, 59, 63
  motor, 20
  prognosis, 224
  sensory, 20
  simple, 19, 20-22
  specific learning disabilities and, 191-193
  specific medicines for, 104, 114
Folic acid, 137
Food, seizure and, 39, 41, 136-139
14 and 6 positive spiking phenomenon, 74, 75
Frostig Developmental Test of Visual Perception, 87

Gelastic seizures, 60
Gemonil, 104, 130
Generalized motor seizure, 13, 15, 25-29
  associated behavioral reactions, 164
  causes, 37
  laboratory diagnosis, 68
  mimicking conditions, 59, 63
  prognosis, 224
  specific medicines for, 104, 114
Generalized motor status, 94
Gesell Developmental Skills Inventory, 84
Gestation seizures, 140
Gilmore Oral Reading Test, 86
Goldman-Fristoe-Woodcock Tests of Auditory Perception and Discrimination, 85
Grand mal seizure, 17, 25-26, *see also* Generalized motor seizure
Grey Oral Reading Test, 86
Group therapy, 144
Gum overgrowth, 131

Hallucinations, 165, 169

Handedness, 47, 190-191
Headache, 61
Head examination
  for bruits, 52, 55
  for pressure, 49
Head-nodding attacks, 29, 63
Head size, 51
Head Start program, 216-218
Head trauma
  examination for, 49
  seizures and, 142-143
Heart, examination, 52-53
Heartbeat, drug dosage and, 98
Helmet, 143
Hemiplegia, 50, 51
Hepatitis, 129
History, components of, 45-47
Hospitalization, 67-68
Housing aid, 218
Hyperactivity, 130, 161-162
  treatment, 171
Hyperventilation, 55-56, 59, 61, 75, 76
Hypsarrhythmia, 76-78
Hysterical seizure, 60, 64, 162

Ictum, 12-13, *see also* Seizure
  brain activity, 14-15
Idiopathic seizure disorder, 35-37
Idiosyncrasy, 129-131
Illinois Test of Psycholinguistic Abilities, 87
Immunization, seizure and, 41
Inborn metabolic disorders, screen for, 70
Individualized education program, 197-198
Infancy, massive spasms of, 29
Infant, jerks and tremors in, 63
Infantile hemiplegic syndrome, 151, 152
Infantile myoclonic spasms, 29, 63
  retardation risk, 194
Infection
  detection, 70, 77
  recurrent seizure and, 101, 102
  seizure and, 38, 53
Inheritance of seizure tendencies, 35-36
Institutionalization, 177-178
Insurance, 204

Intelligence
  deteriorating, 194-195
  range, in epileptics, 194-195
Intelligence tests, 83, 86
Intoxication, 121-125
  chronic, 123-124
  initial, 122-123
  levels of, 121-122
Irritability, treatment, 171
Isotopic brain scan, 80-81, 85

Jackknife seizures, 29
Job training, see Employment

Ketogenic diet, 114, 137-139
Key Math Test, 87

Language examination, 54-55, 85-86, see also Speech
Lasix, 101
Law, rights of epileptic and, 219-220
Learning, drug effects on, 130, 194-195
Learning disabilities, 86, 87, 189-194
Learning problems, 185-200
  behavior and, 186-187
  history, 47
  unrecognized seizures and, 187-188
Left temporal lobe syndrome, 167-169
Lennox Gastaut syndrome, 29
Leukopenia, 128
Librium, 171
Lidocaine, 96, 99
Lightning majors, 29
LSD, seizures and, 136, 154
Lumbar puncture, 71

Magnesium sulfate, 96, 99
Malformation, maternal drug therapy and, 132-133
Mannitol, 101
Marching seizure, definition, 14-15
Marijuana, seizures and, 136, 154
Marriage, 204
Meachem Verbal Language Scales, 85
Mebaral, 104, 106, 130
Medicaid, 213-214

Medical cost assistance, 215
Medical help, 214-216, 218
Medical management, of acute seizure, 96-101
Medicare, 213-214
Mellaril, 171
Memory
  of attack, 13
  erratic, 24
  problems, 187, 193
Meningeal irritation, signs of, 50
Menstruation, seizures and, 39, 139
Migraine headache, 61, 63
Milontin, 105
Minnesota Multiphasic Personality Test, 88
Mirror focus, 15
Mixed seizures
  causes, 37
  prognosis, 223-224
  specific medicines for, 104
Motor Free Visual Perception Test, 87
Motor strip, 20, 21
Mouth ulcers, 128
Movement, abnormal, 62-64
Myoclonic seizure, 28-29
  associated behavioral reactions, 164
  age of onset, 40, 41
  causes, 37
  definition, 17
  prognosis, 224
  specific medicines for, 104, 114
Myoclonic seizure of infancy, brainwave pattern, 76
Myoclonic seizure status, 94
Mysoline, 104, 106, 113-116, 122, 192
  allergic reaction to, 127
  idiosyncratic reactions to, 130, 131
  intelligence deterioration and, 195

Narcolepsy, 60
Neighborhood environment, 179
Nembutal, 96
Neonatal seizure
  causes, 40, 41
  retardation risk, 194
Nephrosis, 129
Neurocutaneous disorder, 52
Neurofibromatosis, 50, 52
Neutropenia, 128

238   Index

Nightmare, 46, 58-59
Nocturnal seizure, 141
Northwestern Syntax Screening Test, 85

Oculomotor apraxia, 63
Oxalodiones, 105

Pancytopenia, 128-129
Papilledema, 49
Paradione, 105
Paraldehyde, 96, 97, 99
Parenthood, 204
Peabody Individual Achievement Test, 86
Peabody Picture Vocabulary Test, 85
PEMA, 107
Pentothal, 96
Petit mal seizure, 17, 26, see also Absence seizure
Petit mal triad, 27
Phenobarbital, 57, 93, 96-99, 106, 107, 112, 113, 124, 192, 195, see also Barbiturates
  allergic reactions to, 127, 128
  idiosyncratic reactions to, 130
  toxicity, 104, 105, 108
Platelet count, 69, 110
Pneumoencephalography, 82-83, 85
Post-ictum brain activity, 13, 15
Posturing, abnormal, 51
Pregnancy
  drug therapy and, 131-133
  seizure and, 39
  seizures during, 133, 139-140
Procaine, 96, 99
Prodrome, 9
  brain activity, 14
Pseudo-collagen disorder syndrome, 127
Pseudo-lymphoma syndrome, 126, 127
Pseudo-rheumatoid syndrome, 127
Psychomotor seizure
  associated behavioral reactions, 164-169
  brain activity, 15
  characteristics, 23-24
  definition, 15, 22
  prognosis, 224

retardation risk, 194
specific medicines for, 104, 114
Psychotic behavior, 169-170
  treatment, 171
Pyridoxine, 137

Rage reaction, 168
Rash, drug-associated, 108, 109, 127, 128
Reading, 189, 191
Recall phenomenon, 147
Recovery, see Post-ictum
Rectal suppository, 98, 125
Reflex sensory seizure
  age of onset, 41
  causes, 39-40
Reinforcement devices, 153
Respiratory support, 96, 98, 99
Reticulocyte count, 69, 110
Reward management, 148
Right temporal lobe syndrome, 167-169
Ritalin, 161
Rorschach Inkblot Test, 89

Salaam spasms, 29
School environment, 179-181
School placement, 195-199
Seconal, 96
Sedatives, seizures and, 136
Seizure, see also specific type
  age of onset, 40-41
  autonomic, 21-22
  causes, 35-42, 46, 101-102
  chronic, causes, 42
  circumstances of, 38-40
  classification, 2, 17-19, 45
  clonic, 26
  course, 41-42
  definition, 9, 13, 16
  diagnosis, steps to, 37, 45
  frequently recurrent, dangers of, 94-95
  heritable tendencies for, 35-36
  induction, 72
  inherited, age of onset, 41
  long, dangers of, 94-95
  major, 17
  major characteristics, 57-58

Index 239

mimics of, 57-65
minor, 17
mixed, 30, 36
multifocal, 30
neonatal, 30
observation of, 55-56
onset, classification by, 18, 19
pathoanatomy, 14
pattern of, changing, 41, 42
primary, 38
recurrent, nerve cell death and, 195
secondary, 38-39
stages, 9-13
timing of, 38-40
tonic, of childhood, 26
types of, 17-33
types of abnormal energy spread in, 14-15
unclassified, 31
unilateral, 29
Seizure, acute, 41-42
  attack types, 93-94
  causes, 41-42
  examination, 48-49
  management, 95-101
Seizure breakthrough
  causes, 101-102
  drug withdrawal and, 117
Seizure management, see also Drug management
  non-drug approaches, 135-155
  ongoing, 103-120
Seizure status, 94
Seizure warning devices, 153
Sentence Completion Test, 89
Serum sickness hypersensitivity reactions, 126-127
Shivering, fever control and, 100
Skull fracture, diagnosis, 49
Skull x-rays, 77-79, 84
Sleep irregularities, seizure and, 39, 141-142
Slingerland Tests, 86
Slossen Intelligence Test, 86
Social maturation tests, 84-85
Social Security benefits, 212-214
Social Security Disability Insurance, 213
Sodium bicarbonate, 100
Sonar encephalogram, 79, 84
Spache Tests of Reading Skills, 86

Spasmus nutans, 63
Speech problems, 47, 188-189
Speech testing, 85-86
Spike pattern, 72, 75, 78
Spike/wave pattern, 75-76, 78
Spinal fluid examination, 71
Sports activities, 201-202
SSI, see Supplemental Security Income
Stanford-Binet Intelligence Test, 86
Staring episodes, 26
  seizure mimics, 61-62
Status epilepticus, 94, 140
Stress management, 135-143
Stroke, 61
Sturge-Weber syndrome, 52
Succinimides, 105
Supplemental Security Income, 212-213
Suppression pattern, 74, 78
Surgical management, 150-152

TAPS, see Training and Placement Service
Team care, components of, 214
Tegretol, 104, 106, 114, 115, 122, 171
  allergic reactions to, 127
  idiosyncratic reactions to, 131
  interaction with other drugs, 115
  laboratory tests during use of, 109
  withdrawal, 119
Temporal lobe foci, specific learning disabilities and, 191-193
Temporal lobe seizure, see Psychomotor seizure
Thematic Apperception Test, 88
Thoughts, abnormal, 24
  seizure mimics and, 58-60
  allergic reactions to, 127
Thrombocytopenia, 128
Tics, 59, 63
Todd's paralysis, 13
Tongue swallowing, 96
Toxemia, 140
Training and Placement Service, 209, 211-212
Tridione, 105, 106, 114-116
  idiosyncratic reactions to, 131
  interaction with other drugs, 115
  laboratory tests during use of, 109
  teratogenic effects, 132

Tuberous sclerosis, 52

Ultrasound studies, 79, 84
University Affiliated Program, 215, 216, 218
Urea, 101
Urinalysis, 70, 110

Valium, 96-99, 105, 112, 114, 115, 117, 171
  allergic reactions to, 127
  interaction with other drugs, 115
Valproate, sodium salt, 96, 105, 114, 115
  allergic reactions to, 127
  interaction with other drugs, 115
  laboratory tests during use of, 109
Ventriculoencephalography, 82-83, 85
Vineland Test of Social Intelligence, 84
Vision, examination of, 54
Vital signs, after acute seizure, 48-49
Vitamin B_6, 137
Vitamin D_3, 137
Vocational aptitude tests, 87-88
Vocational rehabilitation, 210
Vocational Rehabilitation Act of 1973, 209, 217, 219
Vulnerable child syndrome, 174-175

Warning, *see* Aura
Wave pattern, 72, 78
Wechsler IQ tests, 86
WRAT (Wide Range Achievement Test), 86

Zarontin, 105, 106, 113-116, 192
  allergic reactions to, 127
  idiosyncratic reactions to, 131
  interaction with other drugs, 115
  laboratory tests during use of, 109

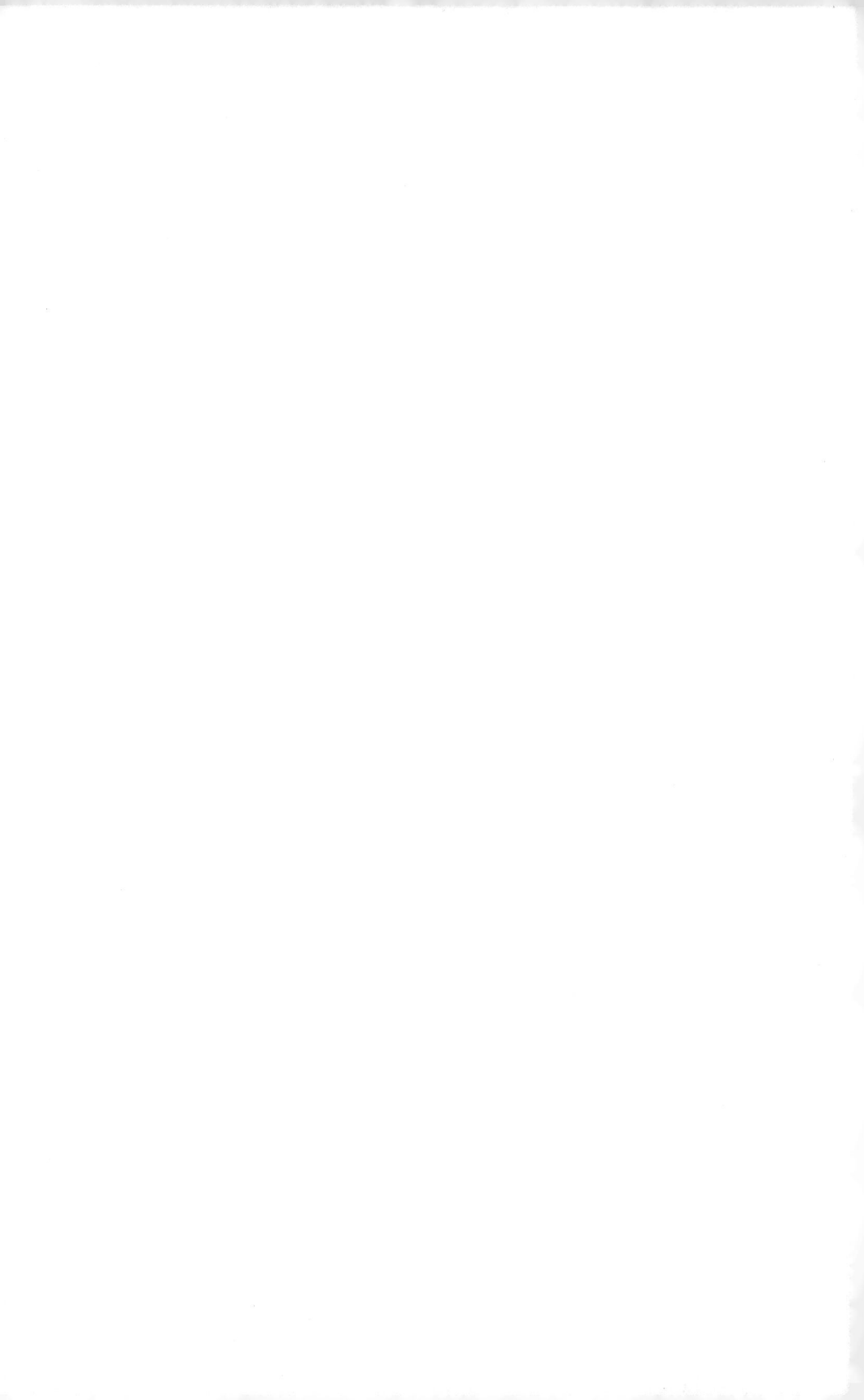